EBURY PRESS

THE CALM PRESCRIPTION

A pioneer of integrative and lifestyle medicine in India, Luke Coutinho has played a crucial role in transforming people's approach to health for over fourteen years. As the Wellness and Lifestyle Champion of Prime Minister Narendra Modi's Fit India Movement, he empowers millions through free educational content, breaking barriers to make health accessible. In a world overloaded with information and marred by confusion, he believes that simplicity is the new luxury.

His philosophy is simple: don't just treat the symptoms—address the root cause. As an author of five national bestsellers, including *Small Wins Everyday*, he shares life lessons to inspire and guide people towards healthier and happier lives. His mission? To educate and make wellness easily available, uncomplicated and empowering for everyone.

ADVANCE PRAISE FOR THE BOOK

'*The Calm Prescription* empowers you to integrate serenity as a non-negotiable part of daily life, rather than a distant aspiration. Luke's effortless practices guide the mind to embrace stillness, so that the body unlocks its natural ability to heal, transforming "dis-ease" into ease'—**B.K. Shivani, motivational speaker, spiritual guide and mentor, Brahma Kumaris**

'An enthusiastic spirit and a happy mind are key signs of well-being, and to lead a happy life, you need a multipronged approach. Luke Coutinho has helped many with his experience in health and wellness. His ability to inspire people to follow good habits and right practices is worth emulating. With this book, may he continue to inspire many on the path of wellness. Love and best wishes'—**Gurudev Sri Sri Ravi Shankar, founder, The Art of Living Foundation**

'Over time, I have come to realize that being CALM allows me to be present in the NOW. And being present is the only way to live every moment to the fullest. So, I consciously work towards finding and staying calm. This book will help people find their calm'—**Vidya Balan, award-winning Indian actor and Padma Shri recipient**

'*The Calm Prescription* is your science-backed guide to healing through stillness, sleep and emotional well-being'—**Ankur Warikoo, entrepreneur and author**

'This book is like a breath of fresh air in a chaotic world. It offers practical wisdom for finding inner peace at an everyday level, which is most crucial. It is more than just a guide; more like an invitation to reclaim our inner peace from within, and I believe it has the potential to transform lives if practised with discipline. A must-read for anyone on the journey of self-discovery and healing, especially in today's world of constant movement and hustle'—**Tamannaah Bhatia, award-winning Indian actor and author**

'Luke's collection of seventy-five evidence-based practices offers something truly precious: accessible pathways to peace that require no special equipment, extensive time commitment or previous experience. His approach resonates deeply with what I've observed throughout my practice—that genuine health begins when we address not just the symptoms of stress but its underlying presence in our daily lives.

'What my patients often don't realize is that grinding teeth at night, tension headaches and accelerated gum inflammation aren't isolated dental concerns—they're physical manifestations of an overwhelmed nervous system seeking release. These subtle signs speak volumes about our body's desperate attempt to find balance in an increasingly unbalanced world.

'This is why *The Calm Prescription* by Luke Coutinho feels like such a necessary companion to holistic healthcare. Between the dental chair and home care routines, I've longed for a resource that addresses what brushing and flossing alone cannot—the fundamental need for inner calm that supports all healing'—**Dr Anil Kohli, BDS, MDS, FDS, RCS and Padma Shri, Padma Bhushan and Dr B.C. Roy Award-winner**

'The strongest organ in our body is our mind. With a strong mind and will, we can achieve the impossible. Part of your health journey has to be emotional health and stress relief. This book will help you return to your mind and to yourself. It aims at healing your body via the untapped power of the mind. This book is so brilliant that you can open to any page and follow the tools for a calmer and readier mind to deal with the restlessness of daily life'—**Dr Nihar Mehta, consultant cardiologist, MBBS, MD (medicine), DNB (medicine) and DNB (cardiology), Sir H.N. Reliance Foundation Hospital, Jaslok Hospital and Breach Candy Hospital, Mumbai**

'Research clearly shows that chronic stress triggers inflammatory cascades and hormonal disruptions that manifest visibly on our skin and silently throughout our bodies. What makes *The Calm Prescription* invaluable is how it translates complex neurobiological concepts into accessible daily practices requiring minimal time commitment.

'Luke has created something remarkable—a wellness resource grounded in science rather than trends, accessible without oversimplification and thorough without overwhelming detail. His personal journey through stress-related health challenges gives these pages an authenticity that resonates deeply.

'As physicians, we aim to equip patients with tools for genuine healing, not just symptom management. *The Calm Prescription* has become that extension of care—a resource I confidently recommend knowing it addresses dimensions of health that brief appointments cannot fully explore'—**Dr Sonali Kohli, MD, senior consultant dermatologist, Sir H.N. Reliance Foundation Hospital, Mumbai**

'In today's era where the hustle culture is the mantra, subconscious stress is affecting an entire generation of professionals. This has a huge impact on health, and as a cancer surgeon, I have seen a huge surge in young cancers. An unhealthy lifestyle is clearly the cause for this. *The Calm Prescription* by Luke is an excellent effort towards empowering everyone with effective techniques to reduce stress and improve productivity and yet maintain a healthy lifestyle. Kudos to him for yet another brilliant endeavour towards mental wellness'—**Dr Ganesh Nagarajan, director, hepatobiliary pancreatic and gastrointestinal oncosurgery, Nanavati Max Institute of Cancer Care**

'In my decades of guiding patients towards healthier lives, I've seen how quietly and deeply stress can wear us down—body, mind and spirit. *The Calm Prescription* by Luke Coutinho offers a radiant path forward. With seventy-five gentle, science-backed practices, it helps restore balance and joy in everyday life. This book is an invitation to live with intention and inner peace' **—Dr Aashish Contractor, director, rehabilitation and sports medicine, Sir H.N. Reliance Foundation Hospital and Research Centre, Mumbai**

'As a cardiologist, I witness the consequences of lifestyle choices daily. Luke's book is not just timely—it's essential. With empathy and depth, he bridges the gap between clinical insight and everyday action. This is more than a book; it's a prescription for lifelong vitality'—**Dr Maulik Parekh, head, Structural Heart Program, Sir H.N. Reliance Foundation Hospital and Research Centre, Mumbai**

'A world overwhelmed by noise, pressure and performance makes *The Calm Prescription* a return to what is essential: the ability to regulate ourselves from within. Emotional intelligence, etiquette and true personal development all begin with the capacity to pause, reflect and respond with presence. Calm is not a luxury—it is a leadership skill, a health imperative and a deeply personal power. Luke's work is a timely and vital reminder that stillness is not the opposite of success—it's the foundation of it.

'Calm is not a passive state—it is a powerful foundation for clarity, emotional regulation and conscious decision-making. In my work as an emotional intelligence and etiquette coach, I've seen time and again that true confidence, grace and leadership cannot emerge from a dysregulated mind or body. The ability to return to calm is what allows us to respond instead of react, to connect instead of control, and to lead from a place of centredness. In a world addicted to urgency, calm is the ultimate strength.

'Calm is the sacred pause between stimulus and response—the space where wisdom lives and resilience is born. It is the gentle anchor in chaos, the quiet confidence beneath composure and the unseen grace behind every thoughtful word or gesture. A regulated nervous system is not only the foundation of emotional intelligence—it is the doorway to fulfilment, connection and presence. When we learn to return to calm, we remember who we truly are'—**Taylor Elizabeth, The Elegance Advisor, internationally acclaimed expert in emotional intelligence and etiquette**

'*The Calm Prescription* is a gentle yet powerful reminder of something yoga has always taught us—that true healing begins within. Luke integrates science and simplicity to help you reconnect with the calm that is your natural state of being. In today's fast-paced world, this book offers a much-needed pause, guiding readers towards balance, emotional wellness and a regulated nervous system. Its holistic approach aligns deeply with the yogic values of self-awareness, mindfulness and inner harmony. I commend Luke for offering such a grounded and accessible path to well-being'—**Hansa Yogendra, director, The Yoga Institute**

'As a doctor with over thirty-five years of practice, I have seen how unresolved stress is a major cause of chronic illnesses. Luke Coutinho's *The Calm Prescription* delivers seventy-five simple, easy-to-adapt practical tips to guide one out of stress and into well-being. A must-read for one and all'—**Dr Anil D'Cruz, MS, DNB, FRCS (hon.), director, oncology, Apollo Hospitals and former president, Union for International Cancer Control, Geneva**

'In cancer care, we rely on advanced therapies—chemotherapy, immunotherapy, precision medicine. But stress is a force that no drug alone can defeat. It weakens immunity, heightens inflammation and may impact every phase of cancer—from risk to recurrence. *The Calm Prescription* by Luke Coutinho is a brilliant companion to modern oncology. Its simple, effective tools help anchor the mind and body in calm—where true healing begins'—**Dr Sachin Trivedi, director, medical oncology, HCG Hospitals Cancer Centre, Mumbai**

'In over three decades of caring for women through every stage of life, I see every day, the intricate link between stress and hormonal health. *The Calm Prescription* by Luke Coutinho presents seventy-five evidence- and experience-based techniques to foster tranquillity and resilience. The book is an invaluable resource for anyone who wants to improve their health through emotional balance. My personal interactions with Luke have always left me energized and thoughtful, and I expect the same for readers of *The Calm Prescription*'—**Dr Nozer Sheriar, gynaecologist, author and women's health advocate**

'Modern gastroenterology is evolving—we now understand that emotional health is intricately linked with digestive well-being. Luke Coutinho's *The Calm Prescription* reminds us of this truth through seventy-five powerful, accessible tools that restore calm and improve overall health. This is more than a book—it's a guide to resilience and gut–brain harmony that I'm proud to endorse'—**Dr Amit Maydeo, Padma Shri awardee, chairman, Institute of Gastrosciences, Sir H.N. Reliance Foundation Hospital, Mumbai and former president, Society of Gastrointestinal Endoscopy of India**

'I've lost count of how many patients with healthy reports still suffered cardiac events—often triggered by prolonged stress. Luke Coutinho's *The Calm Prescription* is a profound reminder that calm is not optional. It is a core prescription for heart protection and longevity'—**Dr Sudhir Pillai, cardiologist, P.D. Hinduja Hospital, Mumbai**

'*The Calm Prescription* by Luke Coutinho is a powerful invitation to step away from the chaos of modern hustle and reconnect with inner peace. Rooted in over fourteen years of science and real-world practice, this book reveals how emotional health and a calm nervous system are the key to true well-being and longevity. With seventy-five simple science-backed tools, it empowers you to shift from stress to calm. No jargon, no equipment, just practical steps you can do any time, anywhere. What exceptional work this has been, by my friend Luke, always offering free and accessible guidance to better health and happiness'—**Vispy Kharadi, 'Steel Man of India', fitness model, sixteen-time Guinness World Record holder and mixed martial arts expert**

'"A diamond is a piece of coal that did very well under stress," Henry Kissinger is reputed to have said.

'The stress—psychological or physiological—will remain so long as the stressors remain, in this highly civilized, urbanized and overambitious world. The stress response of the body is our way to react to a crisis situation, which can be acute or chronic. While the acute response can be the result of polytrauma, overwhelming infections, etc., chronic stress has a far-reaching effect on the body. Therefore, a physiological response can become pathological if the stressors persist. Stress leads to the elaboration of hormones, such as cortisol and adrenaline, which, if prolonged, can affect our sleep and be inimical to the cardiovascular or immune systems. Many cancers are a result of this impaired immune system and inflammatory response.

'We cannot control what happens outside our body, but what happens in our body can be controlled by us. It is not the situation but our reaction and thoughts to it that can define our psychological stress. We must be adept at how we handle this stress.

'In my opinion, the armed forces soldier leads a very stressful life, yet delivers his services in the finest tradition of valour. This is because he has been well-trained in how to handle his stress.

'"Stress is the trash of modern life; we all generate it, but if you do not dispose of it properly, it will pile up and overtake your life," as Danzae Pace has stated.

'*The Calm Prescription* is the finest piece of creative work by Luke Coutinho, in which he elaborates the most simplistic ways you can deal with stress—no gimmicks, no medical jargon, no heavy equipment. This would prove to be everyone's companion and would be handy for a stress-free lifetime.

'As Martin Luther King quoted, "You don't have to see the whole staircase, just take the first step"'—**Dr (Col) Prakash Dave, MBBS, MS, DNB, MNAMS, FAIS, FACS (USA), professor and head, Department of Surgery, Sri Devaraj Urs Medical College, Kolar, Karnataka**

The Calm Prescription

75 Scientific Ways to Create Better Health, Longevity and Happiness

LUKE COUTINHO

EBURY PRESS

An imprint of Penguin Random House

EBURY PRESS

Ebury Press is an imprint of the Penguin Random House group of companies whose addresses can be found at global.penguinrandomhouse.com

Published by Penguin Random House India Pvt. Ltd
4th Floor, Capital Tower 1, MG Road,
Gurugram 122 002, Haryana, India

Penguin Random House India

First published in Ebury Press by Penguin Random House India 2025

10 9 8 7 6 5 4 3 2 1

The statements, opinions and strategies expressed in this book are based on the author's own study and research and the publisher assumes no liability for the same. The publisher and the author provide no warranties of any kind with respect to this book's contents, any line of healthcare, treatment or diet. This book is for informational purposes only and is not intended to diagnose, treat, cure or prevent any condition or disease. It is not intended as a substitute for professional medical advice, diagnosis or treatment, which must be undertaken under the direction of a healthcare provider or physician. Neither the author nor the publisher shall be liable or responsible for any loss or adverse effects allegedly arising from any information or suggestion in this book. While every effort has been made to ensure the accuracy of the information presented, neither the author nor the publisher assumes any responsibility for errors. References are provided for information purposes and do not constitute endorsement of any foods, drugs, medicines or treatments.

ISBN 9780143475941

Typeset in Sabon Lt Pro by MAP Systems, Bengaluru, India

www.penguin.co.in

Contents

Foreword by Dr Jonathan Fisher xv
Introduction xix
Finding the Harmony Within xxiii

Part 1: Foundations of Calm and Wellness

Understanding Homoeostasis: The Body's Balancing Act 3
Embracing Bio-Individuality 9
Unpacking Suppressed and Repressed Emotions 15
The Power of Expression: Releasing Suppressed Emotions for Healing 25
Understanding the Nervous System for a Healthier Life 30

Part 2: 75 Simple Ways of Moving from SNS to PNS

1. Cyclic Sigh/Physiological Sigh 41
2. Wind Chimes 44
3. Go Slump Dump Pump 48
4. Listening to Birdsongs 54
5. Embracing Imperfections 58
6. Lighting a Candle 64
7. Chanting/Humming 68

8. Cold/Hot Therapy 71
9. Massage 76
10. Pets 81
11. Engage Your Senses Consciously 85
12. Make Light of a Situation 90
13. Giving Back and Service 93
14. Grounding Exercises/Barefoot Connections/Walks 97
15. A Warm Cup of Tea, Soup or Coffee 102
16. The Power of a Hug 106
17. Memories and Recalling Happy Moments 111
18. Raising Our Vibrations 115
19. Cloud Gazing 119
20. Decluttering Your Space 123
21. Gargling 127
22. Salt Lamps 129
23. The Half-Salamander 132
24. Limiting Caffeine Intake 134
25. Sitting in Silence 138
26. Warm Bath/Feet Soaking (Epsom Salt Baths) 142
27. Limiting Multitasking 146
28. Mindful Breathing Breaks/Unplanned Pauses 151
29. Stargazing 155
30. Engaging in Artistic Expression 159
31. Restorative Yoga Poses 163
32. Visualization and Guided Imagery 166
33. Positive Affirmation or Autosuggestions 170
34. Smart Fasting 175
35. Thought Checks, Pauses to Challenge and Reframe Negative Thoughts 180
36. Using Food as Medicine 185
37. Limiting Junk, Packaged, Processed and Ultra-Processed Foods 189
38. Deep and Slow Breathing 194
39. Spending Time in Nature 199
40. The Joy of Anticipation 204
41. Slowing Down 208

42. Intimacy, Lovemaking, Orgasms and the Afterglow 213
43. Practising Smiling 218
44. Bonfire/Sitting by a Fireplace 222
45. The Power of Manifestation 226
46. Praying and Wishing Others Well 233
47. Yawning 237
48. Mindful Body Scan 239
49. Morning Routines 241
50. The Gift of Deep Sleep 247
51. Journalling Your Thoughts and Emotions 255
52. Dance Break 258
53. A Tech-Free Day 261
54. Practising Advanced Gratitude 264
55. Staying Present During Your Daily Commute 268
56. Use Calming Scents/Aromatherapy 270
57. Singing 273
58. Sunlight 276
59. Breath Counting 280
60. Create a Nature Sounds Playlist 283
61. Limiting Alcohol 286
62. Deep Conversations 289
63. Following Your Passion 292
64. Movement and Exercise You Enjoy 294
65. The Art of Connection 299
66. Appreciation for Self and Others 303
67. Unplugging to Reconnect 307
68. Cultivating Mindfulness 311
69. Finding Moments of Joy and Laughter Daily 315
70. Crying 321
71. The Power of Meditation 325
72. The Science Behind Music 332
73. Sound Therapy 338
74. Focused Reading for Relaxation 343
75. The Gut–Brain Axis 348

Case Studies 355
Acknowledgements 359

Foreword

It has been a great privilege to know Luke Coutinho and witness his extraordinary impact on so many lives. I still remember our first meeting in San Francisco, where we connected instantly, over shared passions for health, holistic wellness and the vital role of lifestyle in healing. As one of India's foremost health influencers and a global thought leader in wellness, Luke embodies a commitment to well-being, grounded in science and fuelled by a deep sense of purpose.

From the beginning, what struck me most about Luke was his holistic approach to wellness, one that transcends the conventional focus on symptoms alone and recognizes the mind, body and spirit as a complete, interwoven system. Luke's understanding of health goes beyond the basics of diet and exercise, reaching into emotional well-being and spiritual balance. His approach aligns closely with my beliefs as a cardiologist: that health and healing cannot be compartmentalized, but must embrace every dimension of our being. This alignment in our perspectives has led to many profound discussions, inspiring us to expand our work to touch more lives.

Luke graciously invited me to join him as a guest on his podcast, *The Luke Coutinho Show*, where he brings together global leaders to inspire others to live healthier and more fulfilling lives. Each conversation with him has only deepened my admiration for his vision. I have been moved by Luke's steadfast dedication to helping others understand that health is about creating harmony—between body and mind, in our relationships and within our communities. His vision and determination to make a difference extend beyond his work; they are a gift to all who come into his orbit. His dedication to the well-being of others is truly a message for our time, where calmness, resilience and meaningful connections are not luxuries but necessities.

In *The Calm Prescription*, Luke shares transformative insights gleaned from over a decade of guiding thousands of patients through life's greatest challenges. His emphasis on calmness and emotional balance is timely. The relentless pace of our lives, combined with constant demands on our attention and energy, has left many struggling to find an equilibrium. Luke understands deeply that we need to learn how to cultivate calmness from within to thrive amidst today's pressures.

The foundation of this book lies in the role of the parasympathetic nervous system (PNS)—a system essential for relaxation and recovery—and its impact on everything, from immunity and cellular repair to emotional resilience. He shows readers how to shift from constant alertness to deep calmness through approachable explanations and practical techniques. This book offers practical advice and a call to rediscover the transformative power of calmness, which, as research increasingly shows, has profound effects on our health, relationships and overall happiness.

One of the book's most compelling sections is Luke's emphasis on sleep and emotional health as the pillars of vitality. I have seen, first-hand, in my practice, the toll that poor sleep and unmanaged stress take on the heart, in all its dimensions. His guidance on prioritizing sleep and managing emotions, which are too often sidelined in discussions about health, is refreshing and essential. Luke brings a refreshing perspective to calmness, sleep and emotional wellness as the cornerstones of vibrant health, offering practical strategies to help each of us find our way back to the centre.

In addition to covering health's physical, emotional and spiritual pillars, Luke also emphasizes the importance of bio-individuality. This idea—that each of us is unique in our health needs and responses—resonates deeply with my experiences in medicine. There is no one-size-fits-all approach to health; what nourishes one person may not be suitable for another. This principle is woven throughout *The Calm Prescription*, as Luke reminds readers to honour their needs and create a lifestyle supporting their unique wellness paths.

I am particularly inspired by Luke's dedication to accessible, practical advice. In this book, he provides actionable steps for everything—from breathing techniques to daily routines that help activate the PNS. One powerful example is the 'cyclic sigh', a simple breathing exercise that can be used anywhere to reduce stress and bring a sense of calm. These small tools, rooted in both science and ancient wisdom, are designed for real people with real lives, showing that wellness need not be overwhelming or complicated. This focus on simplicity and accessibility makes *The Calm Prescription* a book that can serve as a lasting resource for readers at every stage of their wellness journey.

This book is an invitation to join Luke on a journey that transcends traditional approaches to wellness. He guides us through the profound science of calm and balance, offering tools to change lives and reminding us that health lies in achieving inner peace and resilience. Luke's voice, which is always compassionate, speaks to each reader as a trusted friend, gently guiding them towards greater self-awareness and well-being.

Throughout my journey as a cardiologist, I've come to believe that health is not just about the absence of illness but about the presence of vitality, resilience and a deep connection with oneself, others and the world around us. Luke's work is a testament to this broader understanding of health, and *The Calm Prescription* serves as both a guide and a call to action. This book will be an invaluable companion for anyone seeking to reclaim their vitality, find inner balance or understand the vital importance of calmness.

Luke's teachings could not be more relevant today as we face unprecedented levels of stress and anxiety. He reminds us that cultivating calmness within ourselves has a ripple effect, positively influencing our families, communities and society. When we cultivate calmness and balance within, we are better equipped to lead lives filled with purpose and compassion and to face life's inevitable challenges with resilience and grace.

With deep gratitude and admiration, I invite you to experience the powerful message in these pages. Luke's work and guidance have inspired me, and I know they will inspire you too.

Warmly,

Dr Jonathan Fisher
author of *Just One Heart: A Cardiologist's Guide to Healing, Health, and Happiness*;
cardiologist;
mindfulness teacher and
organizational well-being leader

Introduction

The Calm Prescription—A Path to True Wellness

I have dedicated my practice to Integrative and Lifestyle Medicine, working closely with individuals facing a range of health challenges, including cancer, diabetes, autoimmune conditions, obesity and hormonal imbalances. Throughout this journey, I have gained deep insights that have reshaped my understanding of health and well-being. While we often focus on nutrition, exercise and dietary habits, I've realized that, at the pinnacle of health lies a foundation just as—if not more—critical than these external factors: sleep and emotional wellness.

In our fast-paced world, where hustle culture often dominates, we frequently undervalue the importance of emotional health and quality sleep. Yet, these two elements serve as the bedrock of overall well-being. When emotional health is compromised, restful sleep eludes us, setting off a cascade of consequences that affect physical health, eating habits and even our motivation to exercise.

Research increasingly supports this perspective. Scientific studies highlight how chronic emotional distress and insufficient sleep disrupt hormonal balance, impair immune function and reduce cognitive performance (Cohen et al., 2007; Walker, 2017). Sleep deprivation has been linked to an increased risk of conditions like obesity, diabetes and cardiovascular disease (Spiegel et al., 1999).

The truth is that we cannot simply treat the symptoms of our health issues; we must address their emotional and psychological roots. Prioritizing emotional health is not a luxury, but a necessity. When we cultivate calmness within, we unlock the body's ability to heal and recover at a cellular level. In a state of calm, our cells function harmoniously, enhancing our resilience and enabling us to face life's challenges more effectively.

In this book, *The Calm Prescription,* we invite you on a transformative journey. Here, we explore how creating calmness can help you reclaim not only your health but also your sense of purpose and vitality. This book offers practical tools, insights and strategies to prioritize emotional health and sleep, guiding you to achieve the tranquillity essential for well-being.

As you turn the pages, you will discover the magic that unfolds when you prioritize calmness. In the stillness, healing begins. The connection between a calm mind and a healthy body is not merely theoretical—it is grounded in science, and supported by top neurologists and experts in integrative medicine. The chapters ahead will inspire you to slow down, reflect and make intentional choices that nurture emotional health and well-being.

Let us take this journey together, shifting our focus from the relentless pursuit of diet and exercise plans that often dominate our lives. Instead, we will concentrate on cultivating our emotional landscape and embracing sleep as a quiet sanctuary for healing and rejuvenation. In this state of calm, we can gather the energy needed to pursue our life goals and ambitions with renewed vigour and passion.

Your journey towards calmness, health and vitality begins here. May *The Calm Prescription* serve as a guiding light on this path.

Every patient consultation we hold covers all pillars of health—cellular nutrition, movement, deep sleep, breath, emotional wellness and the spirit. It is, and always will be, a holistic approach because that's how we are designed—an intelligent system of trillions of cells, with constant communication taking place within us. We are not machines that require mere replacements of parts or a superficial treatment of symptoms; we must address the root cause.

In the following pages, we will explore, in a simple way, the workings of the sympathetic and parasympathetic nervous systems (SNS and PNS), so you can understand what's happening inside and to you. I believe deeply in the gift of understanding. When we truly understand and have a powerful 'why', it becomes a game-changer for our health. We shift from simply being told what to do or relying on motivation, to feeling inspired because the how and why are clear.

Following that, we'll share some of the most effective tools and techniques that have worked for so many patients and practitioners over the last thirteen years. I sincerely hope they work for you as well. Even if just one tool, in this entire book, makes a difference, that may be all you need. Keep in mind the concept of bio-individuality: we are all different and unique, and what works for one person may not work for another—and that's okay.

Be patient and calm; these methods are not like pharmaceuticals that promise an immediate but temporary fix. Instead, they address deeper, long-term solutions.

Teach these principles to your loved ones, your children, your community, schools and anyone who needs them. As life gets tougher, we must build resilience against disease and stress by using these tools and living a lifestyle that supports the demands of our world, jobs and environment.

Finding the Harmony Within

I am 38,000 feet above, with a ground speed of 916 km/hour and an air speed of 574 mph as I write this. Flying over Athens, in this beautiful Emirates A380, I am on my way to Manhattan, New York, where, in the next 13 hours, I have the absolute honour of representing my country, India, at the United Nations General Assembly (UNGA) 100 Disruptors' Summit—We The Planet.

As I reflect on what I will speak about, I am drawn to the connection between the health of the planet and our health as human beings. Sustainable solutions for a better and healthier planet must also contribute to a better and healthier us.

As I think about the commonalities, which I see in the world of healthcare today, my mind keeps returning to a point that's impossible to ignore—**chronic stress has become one of the largest contributors to disease.** Physical, emotional and mental health continue to deteriorate as chronic stress influences our actions and behaviours, affecting not only us but also our planet.

Even as you read this, there is new science evolving every minute around exercise, nutrition, sleep and more. Yet, despite all we know, chronic stress, anxiety, fear and suppressed emotions continue to drive illness across all ages. It manifests in various forms, from autoimmune diseases and depression to obesity, cancer, metabolic syndromes and cognitive decline. It amazes me when I meet people, with farms, who grow their food and follow optimal workout routines. Yet, they struggle with disease due to chronic stress and a dysregulated, out-of-balance mind and body.

It's been thirteen years since I began practising integrative and lifestyle medicine, and only now is the healthcare system starting to look at the body as a whole rather than as a sum of separate parts. The system remains fragmented. Top surgeons, neurologists, cardiologists and oncologists, whom I knew ten years ago—who once dismissed the role of stress in human health—have changed their stance. Today, many of them acknowledge that when they cut open a body, replace a heart or radiate a tumour, they are treating a patient weighed down by accumulated stress.

We see rising numbers of workplace suicides and children/teenagers ending their lives because of the chronic epidemic of stress. Relationships and marriages fall apart, not always due to a lack of love, but because love is lost amidst a myriad of stressors.

The big question is: When will we see medical prescriptions that, beyond the pills, also advise patients to improve their nutrition, work out, sleep better and effectively manage stress?

In my segment at the UNGA summit, I plan to speak not about cellular nutrition, angiogenesis, the immune system, inflammation or the gut microbiome. Instead, I will talk about what we truly need—to slow down, calm down, bring harmony and balance back to our bodies and learn to reconnect with our inner spirit. We need to integrate the mind and body, so they work together for us rather than against us. While nutrition, medicine and exercise are important, a calm body, heart and mind are the foundations of prevention, recovery and a meaningful life.

We are not only what we eat, we are what we eat and absorb. We need to be in the right nervous system mode, whether 'fight and flight' or 'rest-and-digest.' When stuck in the wrong mode, we may think that we're eating healthy, but we're not absorbing most nutrients. Malnourishment, even among those who eat well, is becoming alarmingly common, leading to weak immune systems and other cellular-level problems. When our body needs itself to repair, regenerate or sleep, we cannot do so effectively if we remain in a constant state of fight-or-flight.

I remind every patient, whom I see, about the innate intelligence of the human body—a wisdom that exists within each of us. This intelligence works when the body gets what it needs and exists in a balanced environment. It creates harmony among trillions of cells. This intelligence cannot be found in medicine, supplements or superfoods. We must harness it.

When we create the wrong environment, through insufficient or incorrect nutrients, sedentary lifestyles or overtraining, too much or too little sleep and chronic stress, this intelligence works against us. We can continue to treat symptoms with more chemicals, medicines and superfoods, but true recovery and healing will remain out of reach, unless we adopt the tools and energies needed to manage chronic stress and anxiety better.

Eleven years ago, as I walked through Manhattan, after a day of consultations in coffee shops, I remember stopping outside the United Nations (UN), looking in awe at the flags, and watching people in suits leave the building. I wondered what they talked about and what world decisions were made, and I hoped that, one day, I would get the chance to visit the UN from the inside. I am a firm believer in manifestation—both the good and bad in my life have been manifested. While I am thrilled to be a delegate and a part of the important discussions happening, I hope to, one day, share this message about the need for calmness, slowing down and reducing stress in schools and universities. The younger we teach these tools and the more we emphasize that chronic stress should not be normalized, the healthier we will be, as a society.

Every patient I consult with—or my team does—undergoes a diagnosis beyond their lab reports, doctors' notes, nutrition and exercise routines. We dive deep into their emotions and mental health because we believe everything must work together. All the pieces of the puzzle need to fit for a patient to completely heal and recover.

On a typical day, I see eight to twelve patients, and when I travel or give talks, the number may be lower. However, no matter the circumstance, the common theme in the questions I get and the lifestyle programmes we design is this: **better stress and emotion management.** People must understand that their emotional state determines how well they break down, digest and absorb food. It affects how deeply they sleep, how safely they exercise (stress increases the risk of injury) or even if they choose to work out or skip it. It affects their work performance, relationships, food choices, drinking habits and reliance on recreational drugs or medications.

Deep sleep and emotional stress sit at the top of the paradigm of the integrative and lifestyle medicine model. If we are stressed, we can't sleep. If we can't sleep, it affects how we feel the next day, what we choose to eat and our workout decisions. It's more interconnected than you think. Trillions of cells in the human body function best when there is harmony and balance within. This state of balance is known as homoeostasis—something we must all understand more deeply. How do you move to this state? Let's discuss this together.

Part 1

Foundations of Calm and Wellness

Understanding Homoeostasis: The Body's Balancing Act

What Is Homoeostasis?

Let's begin with an analogy. Imagine your body as a well-organized concert hall, with every musician (your organs, cells and systems) playing in harmony to create a beautiful symphony. Homoeostasis is the conductor of this concert, ensuring that each musician plays at the right pace and volume for the song to stay balanced and sound perfect.

When the temperature outside changes, it's like an unexpected gust of wind blowing through the concert hall, threatening to throw everything off. The conductor (homoeostasis) notices and makes quick adjustments. If it's too hot, your sweat glands kick in; if you are too cold, it starts shivering. If your blood sugar spikes after a sweet treat, it's like one musician suddenly playing too loudly—homoeostasis signals insulin, a musician that knows how to lower the volume, to bring it back down.

Just as a good conductor keeps the music smooth, homoeostasis keeps your body steady, making sure that your body's concert plays on without a hitch!

Homoeostasis is the process by which our body maintains a stable internal environment, despite changes in external conditions.

This state of balance is crucial for our overall health and well-being, as it helps regulate vital functions, such as temperature, pH levels, hydration and electrolyte balance.

Why Is Homoeostasis Important?

Maintaining homoeostasis is essential for several reasons:

- **Optimal Functioning:** Our organs and systems work best within specific ranges. When these ranges are disturbed, we may experience fatigue, discomfort or illness.
- **Survival:** Homoeostasis is vital for survival—without it, our cells cannot function properly, leading to severe health complications.

Research published in *Dialogues in Clinical Neuroscience* emphasizes that prolonged disturbances in homoeostasis can lead to various diseases, including metabolic disorders, cardiovascular diseases and autoimmune conditions (McEwen, 2006).

What Disrupts Homoeostasis?

Several factors can throw our body out of balance:

- **Physical Stressors:** Illness, injury or extreme temperatures can challenge our homoeostatic mechanisms.
- **Psychological Stress:** Emotional turmoil can lead to hormonal imbalances that disrupt homoeostasis.
- **Dietary Imbalances:** Poor nutrition—a diet high in processed foods and low in essential nutrients—can lead to dysregulation of bodily functions.
- **Lack of Physical Activity:** Sedentary lifestyles can affect metabolic rates and body composition, leading to homoeostatic imbalances.

The Connection Between Homoeostasis and Disease

When homoeostasis is disrupted, the risk of various diseases increases. Chronic stress can lead to hormonal imbalances, which may result in conditions like hypertension or diabetes. According to research from *Biological Psychiatry*, prolonged imbalance can also contribute to inflammatory responses, further complicating existing health issues (Miller et al., 2008).

How Do We Restore Homoeostasis? Simple Ways to Achieve and Maintain Homoeostasis

Restoring balance is key to feeling our best. Here are some effective methods:

- **Prioritize Nutrition:** Focus on balanced meals and adequate water intake. Eating whole, nutrient-dense foods helps support the body's natural regulation. Meals rich in fruits, vegetables, lean proteins and healthy fats are shown to improve metabolic homoeostasis (Cena and Calder, 2020).
- **Incorporate Regular Exercise:** Aim for at least 150 minutes of moderate activity weekly. Physical activity promotes cardiovascular health and metabolic balance, reducing stress hormones and enhancing mood (Biddle et al., 2015 and 2016).
- **Practice Mindfulness:** Deep, mindful breathing techniques can activate the PNS, reducing stress and promoting relaxation. Studies indicate that breath work can lower cortisol levels and promote well-being (Brown and Gerbarg, 2005).
- **Ensure Quality Sleep:** Maintain a regular sleep schedule and create a restful sleep environment.
- **Seek Nature:** Spending time outdoors has been linked to reduced stress and improved mood. Nature exposure can enhance mental health, facilitating a return to homoeostasis (Kaplan and Kaplan, 1989).
- **Building and Maintaining Positive Relationships:** This can decrease stress and contribute to emotional well-being.

What Are Some Health Benefits of Sustaining Homoeostasis?

- **Increased Energy:** Balanced systems promote better energy levels throughout the day.
- **Improved Mood:** Stable internal environments contribute to emotional well-being, reducing anxiety and depression.
- **Enhanced Immunity:** A balanced body can better fight off infections and illnesses.

Inspiring Ourselves and Others

Understanding the significance of homoeostasis empowers us to take charge of our health. Sharing knowledge and personal experiences with others can inspire collective action.

- **Community Programmes:** Participate in or initiate programmes focused on nutrition, exercise and mental health.
- **Workshops:** Organize or attend workshops on breath work or nature therapy to spread awareness and practice.

Homoeostasis is not merely a biological concept; it's a philosophy for living well. By recognizing the factors that destabilize our balance and implementing lifestyle changes to promote recovery, we empower ourselves and inspire others to thrive in harmony with our bodies and the world around us.

By embracing a holistic approach and understanding the interconnectedness of our choices, we can protect not only our own homoeostasis but also encourage others on their journey towards balance and health.

Our goal, as human beings, should be to reach, stay in and maintain a state of homoeostasis as often and as long as possible.

However, does this mean we should avoid stress? Should we abandon aspirations or ambitions to work, create and achieve more? We all know that many decisions in life—choices related to our roles, promotions, growth and responsibility—will inevitably come with more stress. So, what do we do?

We aim to make ourselves more bulletproof. What do I mean by that? Let me explain.

The army, navy and air force train every day, whether there is a war or not. Why? Because they need to stay fit, strong and informed. They know their enemies are also getting stronger day by day, and they need to be prepared at all times. If they stop training, they will fail, underperform or potentially collapse in the face of real conflict. Similarly, we must train ourselves to handle stress. We have no idea how much more stress life will throw at us.

Have you ever been in a situation where you thought things couldn't get worse, and then they did? Exactly. This is why we need to become bulletproof—so that we don't collapse, get sick or live in a state of misery and helplessness when life demands more from us.

How do we become bulletproof? Is there a magic pill? No. The bulletproof protocol is simple.

To better handle stress and prevent it from ruining our health and well-being, we need to:

- **Eat well and eat smart.** This is the raw material that your cells use to function.
- **Move more.** Stretch, breathe deeply and train your muscle and aerobic capacity. A weak body and mind are less efficient at handling stress.
- **Sleep deeply.** This allows the body to repair, regenerate, balance hormones and recharge.
- **Practise stress management.** Find ways to lower cortisol and bring yourself back to homoeostasis quickly. The more time we spend in the PNS, the better.

When I speak to my patients or my audience at global events, they often ask me about longevity and what it takes to live longer. While science continues to explore new pills, treatments, red light therapy, cold plunges, saunas and other trends, I like to keep things simple. The more time the human body spends in homoeostasis, in the PNS, the longer we may live.

I emphasize this because many so-called longevity experts forget about something called destiny. It's written—it's *Maktub*. None of us is in control of what might happen to us in the next minute, but since we don't fully understand destiny, we set it aside and focus on the actions we can take to live a healthy, meaningful life.

Each day, our goal should be to create a life that allows us to spend more time in the parasympathetic system and homoeostasis—especially when we're under more stress. The more stress we experience, the more the body and mind need to relax. It's all about balance, just like a sedentary body needs more movement. This balance is the key to becoming truly bulletproof.

Embracing Bio-Individuality

Did you know that no two people, including identical twins, have the same pattern of fingerprints?

What does this say about each of us? **We are all unique bio-individuals.** Can you begin to fathom and imagine the intelligence of the universe and nature? There are billions of unique human creations.

Every human being has a different view, feeling and expression of what love is to them, and how they express it to others.

Some like the opposite sex, some the same.

Some stage 4 cancer patients die, while many live for years in remission.

Some bodies thrive on carbs, while some don't.

Some are fat and protein-efficient, some are not.

Some love money, some see it as a curse.

Some are content with what they have, while others want more.

Some like simplicity, some like complication.

Coffee and tea may be good for many, but not for others.

Some have a peg or two in their nineties, and are happy and healthy, while some start experiencing issues with the liver or addiction problems with alcohol.

Some express love and still you don't feel it, whereas some don't express it, yet you feel it.

Some like intimacy and some don't.

Some have certain ways of lovemaking and expressing love, while others do it differently.

Some relationships thrive, some don't.

Some people heal faster, some don't.

Some manage well with fasting, some don't.

Some kids can manage video games; for others, video games manage them.

The reason our health, relationships and personal growth are at their worst at this point is that society, media, social media, communities, medicine, fitness and spirituality are all trying to put each of us in a box.

It is a one-shoe-fits-all or cookie-cutter approach to control, confuse, sell, make huge profits the wrong way, play with human emotions and induce fear by making you feel inadequate.

When you know that you are intelligently unique, how can comparing, copying others and putting yourself in extreme boxes, fads or regimes ever work for YOU?

The biggest fear of the lobbies will be when humans start to look and connect within and understand that solutions come from within. When they stop you from comparing yourself with others, they stop selling the comforting lie.

Learn, absorb, study, get mentored, but relate all your learning with what your mind, body, heart and soul need. Not because the world, your friends or your social circle is doing it, but because it's meant for you and you are a unique bio-individual with unique means. Not mediocre needs, but unique and powerful needs.

What Is the Essence of Bio-individuality?

The idea of bio-individuality holds that every individual is distinct in their emotional experiences, lifestyle preferences and biological composition. Our body's response to nutrition, exercise, stress and different health interventions are examples of this individuality. Developing individualized approaches to health and well-being requires an understanding of this diversity.

What Does Science Say?

Genetic differences—such as single nucleotide polymorphisms (SNPs)—can significantly influence how individuals metabolize nutrients, respond to exercise and react to stressors (Niforou, Konstantinidou, and Naska, 2020). For instance, genetic predispositions can affect everything from vitamin absorption to the likelihood of developing chronic diseases, indicating a need for personalized nutritional recommendations.

A 2021 study published in *The Journal of Nutrition* highlights that variations in metabolic pathways can lead to different responses to macronutrients (LaBarre, Singer, and Burant, 2021). This evidence supports a personalized approach to nutrition, as what works for one person may not yield the same results for another.

The Pitfalls of Cookie-Cutter Approaches

The traditional 'one-size-fits-all' model in health is like using a generic mould to shape individuals—riddled with limitations. Any plan that disrespects or ignores your bio-individuality often leads to frustration, failure or deterioration. For example, a diet that works well for your friend may prove detrimental to you, and add to feelings of inadequacy and confusion.

Clinical evidence corroborates this. Studies show that standardized approaches—like low-calorie or low-carb plans—have varying rates of success across populations (Sacks et al., 2009). This variance often stems from the complex interplay of genetics, environmental influences and personal preferences.

The Need for Holistic Approaches

A holistic perspective on health recognizes that biological, psychological and social factors intertwine in shaping our well-being. If you need your lifestyle or health plan to work for you, integrating these elements is crucial.

Nutrition: The Individual Plate

Nutrition is a perfect illustration of bio-individuality. Beyond genetics, factors like gut microbiota and personal health history can influence how we assimilate and utilize nutrients. Research by the National Center for Health Statistics (NCHS) emphasizes diverse ways nutrients affect metabolism, highlighting the need for individualized dietary plans based on personal health assessments (Bush et al., 2019).

For example, some individuals thrive on high-carb diets, while others might experience inflammation and weight gain. Thus, understanding one's unique responses to different foods—not by comparison but through personal exploration—can pave the way for optimal nutrition.

Movement: The Personal Journey of Exercise

Exercise, much like nutrition, requires customization. The body responds variably to different types of physical activity. Genetic predispositions can determine an individual's strength, endurance and flexibility (Bouchard et al., 1999).

While one person might thrive on high-intensity training, another may find greater enjoyment and result in gentler, restorative exercises like yoga or Tai Chi. Embracing these differences encourages people to seek activities that resonate psychologically and biologically, promoting consistency and long-term benefits.

Mental and Emotional Health: The Unseen Factors

The complexity of bio-individuality extends into our mental and emotional health too. Yes, socio-economic status and community connections affect well-being. However, our personal experiences shape our emotional states and resilience to stress.

Research shows that personalized mental health approaches are more effective than standardized ones. For instance, cognitive behavioural therapy (CBT), tailored to individual experiences, often yields better results than generic programmes (Hofmann et al., 2012). This reaffirms that seeing a person purely as a symptom or disorder isn't just reductionist; it undermines the multidimensional nature of human health.

Thinking Outside the Box: A Call to Action

Understanding and embracing bio-individuality builds a culture of going the extra mile and exploring what works for you. Think of each individual as a unique constellation of experiences, genetics and preferences.

How Can You Respect This Bio-individuality?

Engaging with healthcare providers, nutritionists and lifestyle coaches, who emphasize personalized care, can empower people to take charge of their health.

Encouraging individuals to experiment with their diets, exercise regimes and mental health practices—each discovery brings you closer to understanding what works best for you.

Building a community that values and encourages individuality creates an environment in which experimentation is safe and supported.

This deep respect for bio-individuality has been the foundation of my practice for the last thirteen years and continues to be so to date.

The Path Forward: Value Individuality

In a world that is quick to categorize and label, it is crucial to recognize the beauty of human diversity. By celebrating bio-individuality, we honour not just our differences but the unique paths we must take to create optimal health.

The science is clear: generic approaches often lead to mediocre results, at best, and frustration, at worst.

In an age where personalized medicine is on the rise, it is time to adopt a holistic model that respects the uniqueness of every individual.

Today, there is ample evidence to support bidding goodbye to cookie-cutter models. Embracing bio-individuality is not just a scientific necessity—it is a moral requirement.

A Collective Journey

As we embark on our health journeys, let's extend our understanding beyond traditional frameworks. Instead of striving for perfection based on societal norms, let's redefine health in personalized, meaningful ways.

By recognizing our unique compositions and paving the way for individually tailored health strategies, we can inspire ourselves, and others, to thrive, thereby encouraging a healthier and more vibrant society where each person embraces their distinct essence.

By shifting the narrative and creating space for bio-individuality, we move closer to a health paradigm that celebrates each person—not only as a number or statistic but as a complex, beautiful organism with a unique story to tell.

Unpacking Suppressed and Repressed Emotions

As humans, we all express emotions that range across the spectrum. These emotions influence our attitudes, actions and general well-being. However, many of us have trouble processing our feelings, whether it's because of social expectations, shame or fear. When this happens, two main outcomes frequently result: **suppressed** and **repressed emotions.**

I see this in my practice, almost every day. One out of three of my patients struggles with suppressed and repressed emotions. However, there's a big difference between the two. And we're going to understand this.

Decoding the Difference between Suppressed and Repressed Emotions

Feelings that we deliberately ignore, or avoid, are known as **suppressed emotions.** For example, to avoid conflict, someone may choose to remain silent during a heated dispute with a loved one, thus suppressing their anger.

Conversely, **repressed emotions** are ones that are inadvertently stored deep inside the mind, frequently as a form of self-defence. When a loved one passes away, for instance, a person may suppress their sadness, thereby cutting off their emotional reaction.

Everyone has some repressed and suppressed emotions, including me. It's human nature. The distinction is that some of us are able to cope with and channel it, while some let it fester deep within, which, over time, can lead to more negative emotions, sickness and disease.

There's enough scientific information showing us the connection between suppressed and repressed emotions with disease.

American bestselling author and professional motivational speaker, Louise Hay, who has given the world several gems, like *You Can Heal Your Life* (1984), speaks about these various connections.

Emotional and Mental Links to Physical Ailments

- **Digestive Issues:** These may stem from resistance to embracing new experiences or a fear of unfamiliar ideas.
- **Throat Discomfort:** Often connected to suppressed emotions, difficulty expressing oneself or unspoken hurt.
- **Back Pain:** Could be rooted in a lack of emotional or financial support, feelings of guilt or holding back love and care.
- **Vision Problems:** Might reflect dissatisfaction with one's life or a reluctance to face the past, present or future.
- **Knee Pain:** Associated with rigidity, pride or difficulty adapting and being flexible in life.
- **Mouth Issues:** Can signify a resistance to fresh perspectives, a closed mindset or deeply held opinions.
- **Colon Concerns:** Often linked to an emotional struggle in letting go of the past or clinging to outdated beliefs.
- **Leg Problems:** May indicate fear or hesitation in progressing towards the future.
- **Headaches:** Frequently connected to self-criticism, emotional stress or inner conflict.
- **Weight Gain:** Sometimes a form of self-protection, a response to emotional insecurity or a way to compensate for feelings of loss or fear.

- **Constipation:** Tied to difficulty in releasing emotional baggage or a tendency to hoard—emotionally or materially.
- **Cancer:** Often reflects deep emotional wounds, long-standing resentment and a sense of hopelessness or emotional defeat.
- **Stiffness in the Body:** May mirror mental inflexibility or attachment to outdated patterns and beliefs.
- **Swelling:** Indicates emotional stagnation, suppressed grief or blaming others for one's situation.
- **Tumors:** Suggest holding on to old emotional pain, unresolved grudges or past traumas for extended periods.

I often meet patients who come to me and say, *'Luke, I know why I have cancer. I know why I had this stroke.'* They speak of deep-seated emotions—intense rage, bitterness, guilt, anger, betrayal and hurt—that they have carried for years.

The human body is equipped with incredible tools for self-healing. However, a pill alone cannot fix everything. This reliance on medications has contributed to today's high rates of chronic illness, as many believe that a pill can solve everything—from psychological issues to cancer, diabetes and heart disease. Of course, medicine has its place and can be life-saving. But we must also ask, why are you sick in the first place? True healing comes from addressing the root causes.

Many people today are unwell because they harbour unprocessed, festering emotions. We know that anger can increase the risk of heart attacks and cardiac events. Most people with high blood pressure, in fact, live with repressed emotions.

Let's talk about suppressed emotions with an example.

Imagine you dislike your boss and have a strained relationship with them. Today, they've called you in for a feedback session—on them. They're the person who holds power over your promotions, so, although you want to be honest, and say, 'You're biased, rude, dismissive of work-life balance, egoistic and unwilling to listen,' you're hesitant. With appraisals around the corner, you feel you can't speak your truth. Instead, you tell them, 'Everything's going well; you're a great boss,' while your real feelings stay bottled up.

Now, you go home with these pent-up emotions. Maybe you vent to a friend, or hit the gym, letting loose on a punching bag while imagining your boss's face on it.

When we suppress an emotion, we essentially 'shelve' it temporarily. We may revisit it later through venting, gossiping or more constructive outlets like journalling, talking to a trusted friend or exercising. This is what we'd call healthy suppression: we set aside the emotion temporarily but return to process it in a way that doesn't harm us.

Unhealthy suppression, however, happens when we avoid addressing the root of the emotion entirely. Instead, we might turn to coping mechanisms like drinking, smoking, doing drugs or compulsive shopping. These activities distract us but don't allow us to deal with the emotion—and the original issue remains unaddressed, often intensifying over time.

What Is Repression and Why Is It Worse Than Suppression?

Repression is the unconscious blocking of distressing emotions, memories or experiences. Imagine a young girl who suffers abuse by a close relative and courageously turns to her parents for help. Instead of receiving support, she's told, 'Don't speak of this. No one will marry you; you'll be shunned.' Her plea for comfort is dismissed, and she is pressured to stay silent. To cope, her mind begins to block out this trauma, pushing the memory and emotions into her subconscious because she is not allowed to express or process them.

This leads to deep-rooted fears and distorted beliefs like, 'No one will believe me,' or 'People will think it was my fault.' Over time, she unconsciously represses this memory, disconnecting from the event and the emotions tied to it. Repressed emotions remain within us, buried but not gone, often surfacing unexpectedly through physical or emotional distress.

There's evidence that repressed emotions can manifest in physical ways. One remarkable example comes from Cambodia, wherein women were forced to witness soldiers killing their families. Many developed blindness as a psychological defence—an extreme reaction to avoid seeing the trauma unfold. Yes, they induced blindness to cut out that scene in front of them completely. This is the power of the human mind. The ability to block out overwhelming emotions and memories is well-documented in medical literature.

Repressed emotions often correlate with conditions like high blood pressure, obesity and even cancer. Though there are many contributing factors to these illnesses, repressed emotions can be a hidden trigger. When something stirs up these buried emotions—a familiar sight, smell or situation—people may feel sudden, unexplained anger or anxiety. Often, this response stems from an unprocessed, repressed memory, perhaps from childhood or a toxic relationship, surfacing without their conscious understanding.

If unaddressed, repressed and suppressed emotions can become one of life's biggest barriers, limiting our ability to heal, grow and live fully.

Why Do These Suppressed/Repressed Emotions Matter?

Suppressed and repressed emotions matter deeply because they have a profound impact on our health, down to the cellular level. Research has shown that our emotions directly affect our physical well-being, making it essential to acknowledge and care for our emotional health.

We are all born with traits like anger, jealousy, envy and bitterness. No one escapes these emotions, not even experienced meditators or spiritual practitioners. When

I speak with my *Vipassana* and yoga teacher friends, who have dedicated their lives to inner peace, they too face emotions of anger, jealousy, rejection and abandonment. Life in today's chaotic, fast-paced world, filled with stressors and constant triggers, often causes these emotions to arise. Yet, many of us instinctively push them down, storing them within.

Health—good or bad—begins at the cellular level. Every thought, feeling and emotion resonates throughout our trillions of cells. Think about how you feel physically when anger, jealousy, rejection, resentment or bitterness arise. Your body tightens, contracts and feels heavy, the opposite of how it feels when you're happy and relaxed. Every one of those trillions of cells absorbs that negative vibration, which affects cellular health and drains energy meant for your brain, skin, liver, kidneys and other organs.

Unprocessed emotions and unresolved trauma can lead to chronic health issues, including cancer, autoimmune diseases and inflammation. By addressing these emotions, we can begin to clear the way for better health and prevent them from becoming underlying drivers of chronic disease.

The Relationship Between Emotions and Health and the Science Behind It

The impact of suppressed and repressed emotions on physical health is profound. A growing body of research demonstrates a clear connection between our emotional experiences and various medical conditions. The role of emotional health is increasingly being recognized as a crucial factor in both preventive and recovery-based healthcare.

- Studies indicate that suppressing emotions can lead to physical ailments by triggering harmful physiological responses. Dr Gabor Maté, a renowned physician and author of *When the Body Says No*, emphasizes how unresolved emotional conflicts can manifest as physical illness (Maté, 2003).

- Research published in *Psychological Bulletin* highlights a strong correlation between emotional distress and the immune system, showing that chronic emotional suppression can lead to immunosuppression (Segerstrom et al., 2004). This weakened immune system makes individuals more vulnerable to conditions such as autoimmune diseases, diabetes and cancer (Slavich and Irwin, 2014).

Anger and the Liver

Anger is not just an emotional reaction; its repression can harm our physical health. Traditional Chinese medicine often links anger to the liver, and chronic frustration or resentment can manifest in liver-related issues such as fatty liver disease or hepatitis. Research supports this, showing that individuals with chronic stress including suppressed anger have higher levels of liver enzymes (Xu et al., 2022).

Grief and the Lungs

Grief can also significantly affect respiratory health. Individuals grieving a loss may experience physical symptoms like shortness of breath or chronic coughing. This in turn may exacerbate conditions such as asthma or chronic obstructive pulmonary disease (COPD) (Mughal et al., 2023).

Financial Insecurity and Back Pain

Financial stress can lead to heightened anxiety, which often manifests as chronic back pain. Research shows a strong connection between financial worries and increased musculoskeletal pain (Rios and Zautra, 2011) as psychological stress causes muscle tension, resulting in physical discomfort.

Low Self-Esteem and Multiple Sclerosis

Suppressed emotions, particularly low self-esteem, have been linked to autoimmune diseases like multiple sclerosis (MS). Dr Nancy Klimas, a leading expert in chronic fatigue syndrome and autoimmune disorders, notes how emotional stress can trigger immune dysregulation and lead to disease (Klimas et al., 2021).

The Role of Emotional Expression

The power of emotional expression cannot be overstated. Dr James Pennebaker, a distinguished psychologist, found that expressive writing—encouraging individuals to articulate their thoughts and feelings—can significantly improve both mental and physical health outcomes (Pennebaker, 1997). Those who engage in this practice often report lower anxiety, improved immune function and greater emotional clarity.

Expressing emotions retrains the mind and body, releasing pent-up feelings that, if left unaddressed, contribute to disease. Acknowledging and processing emotions through journalling, therapy or open communication help build resilience and foster healing.

The Immune System Connection

Suppressing emotions doesn't just impact our psychological well-being; it can also compromise our immune system. Research identifies a bi-directional relationship between emotional states and immune responses, showing that suppressed emotions can lead to inflammation and weaken immunity (Holt-Lunstad et al., 2010).

For example, chronic stress, often resulting from unexpressed emotions, elevates cortisol levels. When cortisol remains persistently high, it impairs T-cell function and immune regulation, increasing the risk of illnesses such as diabetes, inflammatory conditions and even cancer (Kiecolt-Glaser et al., 2002).

How Emotional Suppression and Repression Are Connected With Chronic Diseases

- Chronic stress from unresolved emotions increases inflammation, a common factor in heart disease, diabetes and cancer.

- Chronic stress can dysregulate the immune system, leading to autoimmune diseases (e.g., rheumatoid arthritis) and weakened immune responses, affecting cancer progression.
- Psychological stress affects the nervous and immune systems, increasing inflammation and disease risk.
- Stress-induced cytokine production promotes inflammation and disease.
- Trauma can cause epigenetic changes that affect gene expression and disease susceptibility. These changes can be passed onto future generations.
- Trauma-related mental health issues, like depression and anxiety, can worsen physical health. Psychological distress can lead to unhealthy behaviours, increasing disease risk.
- Chronic stress promotes tumour growth and metastasis through inflammation and DNA damage.
- Chronic stress triggers autoimmune responses through inflammation and hormonal imbalances.
- Stress-induced brain inflammation increases the risk of cognitive decline and neurodegenerative diseases.

The Path to Healing: Embracing the Calm Prescription

To embrace the calm prescription, we must first recognize the importance of expressing these emotions. Here are actionable steps to promote both emotional and physical healing:

- Techniques like meditation or yoga help cultivate self-awareness and encourage individuals to connect with their emotions.
- Writing about your thoughts and feelings regularly allows for the processing of emotions and greater emotional clarity.
- Engaging with trained professionals—such as psychologists, counsellors or life coaches—provides a safe space to explore and process emotions.

- Surrounding yourself with a supportive community fosters connection and makes it easier to express emotions authentically.
- Regular exercise not only relieves stress but can also serve as a medium for emotional expression.

A Journey Towards Emotional Freedom

The journey towards emotional freedom is crucial for our mental, emotional and physical well-being. By unpacking suppressed and repressed emotions, we dismantle the barriers that prevent us from achieving true health.

As we move from avoidance to acceptance, we embrace a life characterized by honesty, empathy and resilience. Each emotion is a vital piece of our unique human experience, deserving of acknowledgment and expression.

In honouring our emotional landscapes, we empower ourselves with the ultimate prescription for a calm, vibrant and healthier life.

The Power of Expression: Releasing Suppressed Emotions for Healing

Emotions are not just fleeting feelings; they are powerful messengers that reflect our inner experiences, deeply held beliefs and values. Suppressing emotions or burying them deep within can result in far-reaching physical and psychological consequences. Whether it is unaddressed anger, grief or shame, when emotions are left unchecked, they create a ripple effect, impacting both mind and body.

The mind-body connection is a growing area of study, with a strong emphasis on how suppressed emotions can manifest as physical ailments. Scientists, psychologists and medical professionals agree: our emotional state plays a significant role in our overall health. Chronic illnesses, anxiety, depression, autoimmune disorders and even cancer have been linked to unresolved emotional trauma. In this chapter, we'll explore the importance of expressing emotions, the science behind it and how you can take steps to release what you've been holding inside.

The Mind-Body Connection and Suppressed Emotions

Leading experts in psychosomatic medicine—such as Dr Gabor Maté—argues that emotions and physical health are intertwined. In his book, *When the Body Says No*, Maté explores how emotional repression can contribute to chronic illnesses. He suggests that individuals who suppress emotions, like anger or sadness, may be at a higher risk of developing conditions such as autoimmune disorders, heart disease and cancer. When emotions are ignored, they often manifest physically, either in the form of tension headaches, digestive problems or fatigue.

Research published in *Psychosomatic Medicine* supports this idea, demonstrating that individuals with a tendency to suppress emotions show increased markers of inflammation and oxidative stress in the body—two key processes that contribute to the development of chronic illnesses like heart disease and diabetes.

Renowned psychiatrist Dr Bessel van der Kolk, author of *The Body Keeps the Score*, emphasizes the importance of releasing trapped emotions to prevent trauma from taking root in the body. He highlights how trauma survivors often carry the physical imprints of emotional pain in their bodies, leading to issues like chronic pain and fibromyalgia. 'Our bodies hold onto the emotional experiences we don't process,' he notes, adding, 'and this can create a cascade of physical problems.'

Why Expressing Suppressed Emotions Matters

1. Psychological Relief

One of the most well-known studies on emotional expression, led by Dr James Pennebaker, found that people who engage in expressive writing about their suppressed emotions experienced improved mental health and well-being. This study, published in *Psychological Science,* highlighted how emotional writing helps people process traumas and unburdens the mind. By engaging in reflective writing, individuals can come to terms with their experiences, gaining both psychological and cognitive relief.

2. Physical Health Benefits

Dr Gabor Maté suggests that emotional suppression contributes to immune system dysregulation. His work emphasizes how the act of emotional expression can serve as a release valve, reducing the body's inflammatory responses, which can lead to chronic illness when left unchecked.

3. Social Support and Connection

A study from the *American Psychological Association* showed that sharing emotions with trusted friends or in therapeutic settings deepens social connections and provides significant stress relief. This social support can act as a buffer, reducing the health risks associated with stress and emotional suppression.

A Step-by-Step Plan for Emotional Expression

Step 1: Self-Reflection and Awareness

Action: Take time, daily, for introspection. Ask yourself:

- What emotions do I suppress most often?
- Do certain memories or experiences trigger physical sensations?
- How do I react when uncomfortable emotions arise?

Method: Start with journalling. Let your thoughts flow without judgement. Write freely about your feelings and physical sensations.

Step 2: Identify Your Suppressed Emotions

Action: List the significant events in your life that you feel are unresolved. It could be childhood trauma, break-ups or the loss of a loved one.

Method: As you create this list, categorize each event by the primary emotion associated with it—anger, sadness or fear. Pay attention to any physical symptoms that accompany these emotions, such as stomach pain, headaches or fatigue.

Step 3: Start Expressing Through Writing

Action: Pick one of the emotions or events identified in Step 2 and write about it.

Method: Write freely, for 15–20 minutes, about your experience without censoring yourself. This 'free writing' allows you to unlock emotions you may not even realize you've been suppressing.

Step 4: Find Your Voice

Action: Express your emotions in creative ways or share them with someone you trust.

Method:

- **Art:** Use drawing, painting or even music to visualize or express your emotions.
- **Support Groups:** Speak to a counsellor or join a support group. These spaces are designed for sharing deep, personal experiences and emotions.

Step 5: Incorporate Mindfulness Practices

Action: Use mindfulness techniques to stay connected to your emotions in a healthy way.

Method:

- **Meditation:** Focus on breathing and body awareness to stay present with your emotions.
- **Breath Work:** Deep breathing exercises can help release emotional tension stored in the body.

Step 6: Seek Professional Support

Action: Seek the guidance of a therapist or counsellor if the emotions feel too overwhelming to handle alone.

Method: Techniques such as Eye Movement Desensitization and Reprocessing (EMDR) and CBT have been shown to be effective in helping individuals process deep-seated emotional trauma.

The Mind-Body Prescription: Sustaining Emotional Expression

- **Daily Check-ins:** Set aside a few minutes each day to reflect on your emotional state and how it manifests in your body.
- **Celebrate Progress:** Each step towards emotional expression is a victory. Acknowledge your efforts and growth as you work through suppressed feelings.
- **Balance with Gratitude:** Keep a gratitude journal to acknowledge positive emotions. Balancing difficult emotions with appreciation for the good can help you maintain emotional equilibrium.

The process of releasing suppressed emotions may seem daunting, but the benefits are clear—better mental health, improved physical well-being and deeper, more authentic relationships. Emotions are not meant to be buried; they are designed to be felt, processed and expressed.

Let go of what weighs you down and embrace the healing that comes from expressing your emotions. The road to emotional expression is one that leads to peace, authenticity and true health.

Understanding the Nervous System for a Healthier Life

In our journey to live a healthy, fulfilling life, few systems are as crucial—and as often misunderstood—as the nervous system. The nervous system, a complex web of communication pathways, governs everything—from our heartbeats to our ability to face and handle stress. Central to this intricate network is the Autonomic Nervous System (ANS), which acts like a two-lane highway that drives our responses to life's challenges and opportunities. This system consists of two main branches: the Sympathetic Nervous System (SNS) and the PNS. These two systems work in harmony, each serving a unique and critical role in maintaining balance and ensuring survival.

The Sympathetic Nervous System: Fight, Flight or Freeze

Imagine you're suddenly confronted with a threat—an unexpected danger or high-pressure situation. This is when the SNS leaps into action, flooding your body with adrenaline and preparing you to either stand your ground, run for safety or freeze momentarily to assess the situation. This response, often termed the 'fight, flight or freeze' reaction, has been our ally since the dawn of humanity, enabling us to survive in a world filled with predators and hazards.

What Happens When the SNS Is Activated?

Activation of the SNS results in a powerful cascade of physiological changes, allowing the body to respond to stress efficiently:

- **Increased Heart Rate:** The heart accelerates, pumping blood more rapidly into the muscles and brain. This prepares your body for physical action—whether to confront danger or make a swift escape.
- **Dilated Pupils:** Your pupils widen, allowing more light to enter and sharpening your vision so you can better assess potential threats.
- **Quickened Breathing:** Your breathing becomes faster and shallower, supplying oxygen to muscles more efficiently.
- **Heightened Alertness:** The brain releases neurotransmitters, like adrenaline and norepinephrine, enhancing focus and decision-making speed.

These changes are vital for immediate survival. Blood flow is diverted from less critical functions, such as digestion and reproduction, to the muscles, brain and other areas crucial for rapid action. For short bursts, the SNS is not only beneficial but also necessary—it's how our ancestors escaped predators or faced hostile encounters.

The Extraordinary Feat of Hysterical Strength

One of the most captivating examples of the SNS in action is the phenomenon known as hysterical strength—a sudden, superhuman burst of energy often witnessed in life-threatening situations.

A widely cited example of this occurred in the 1980s, involving a mother who exhibited an incredible act of strength to save her child. Her young son was pinned under a car following a minor accident. In the heat of the moment, with her son's life in immediate danger, she somehow managed to lift the car just enough to free him. This was not a story of trained muscle or extraordinary physical fitness; it was an ordinary woman harnessing extraordinary power.

In that split second, her body went into full SNS overdrive—her heart was racing, every muscle was firing at peak capacity and adrenaline was surging through her bloodstream. Blood flow was rerouted to her limbs, allowing her the strength to perform a feat that would have been impossible under normal circumstances. This sudden surge of energy—often described as the power of 'ten men'—is a vivid illustration of how the SNS prepares us to handle extreme stress and danger, summoning reserves we didn't even know we had.

However, while the ability to summon such strength is astonishing and even life-saving, it's not without a cost. Prolonged or chronic activation of the SNS can strain the body, leading to health issues if the system remains on high alert for too long.

What Happens When the SNS Is Overused?

SNS is indispensable in the face of real danger, but in today's world, threats are often psychological rather than physical. Instead of confronting wild animals or natural disasters, we're more likely to face work deadlines, social pressures and past traumas. Yet, the body reacts the same way. Over time, chronic activation of the SNS—being stuck in a prolonged state of 'fight-or-flight'—can cause detrimental effects to our health:

- **Digestive Issues:** Blood is continually directed away from the digestive tract, impairing nutrient absorption and leading to gut-related problems.
- **Sleep Disruption:** Elevated cortisol and adrenaline levels interfere with the body's natural sleep cycles, causing insomnia or poor-quality sleep.
- **Immune System Suppression:** Chronic stress compromises immune function, making the body more vulnerable to infections and illness.

- **Increased Inflammation:** Persistent SNS activation can cause systemic inflammation, linked to conditions like cardiovascular diseases, diabetes and autoimmune disorders.

Real-life examples are everywhere: the executive who feels pressure before a major presentation, the student with butterflies in their stomach during exams or even the sudden surge of adrenaline while narrowly avoiding a car accident. These situations trigger the SNS, temporarily sacrificing long-term health for short-term survival. The key is not to suppress the SNS but to ensure it is activated only when genuinely necessary.

The PNS: Rest, Digest and Heal

In contrast to the high-alert state of the SNS, the PNS is like a soft reset button—a calming counterbalance that allows the body to rest, recover and rejuvenate. Often called the 'rest-and-digest' system, the PNS encourages relaxation and restoration, enabling the body to repair itself and function at its best.

What Happens When the PNS is Activated?

When the PNS takes charge, the body's physiology shifts from stress mode to relaxation mode:

- **Heart Rate Decreases:** The heart slows down, allowing the body to relax.
- **Digestive Processes Activate:** Blood flow returns to the stomach and intestines, promoting effective digestion and nutrient absorption.
- **Immune Function Strengthens:** The body focuses on healing and recovery, fortifying defences against illness.
- **Hormonal Balance:** Cortisol and adrenaline levels drop, while hormones related to well-being, like oxytocin and serotonin, are released.

Activating the PNS helps maintain equilibrium, lowers stress and supports long-term well-being. This is why moments of calm and relaxation—like taking a deep breath, engaging in gentle yoga, spending time in nature or practising gratitude—are so crucial for both physical and mental health.

Why the Balance Between the Two States Matters

Both the SNS and PNS are essential; they are not adversaries but partners in a delicate dance that keeps us healthy and capable. The SNS allows us to face emergencies and challenges, while the PNS enables us to recover and thrive once those challenges have passed. Problems arise not from activating the SNS, but from remaining stuck in that mode for too long. This chapter aims to guide you in recognizing when to switch from the 'fight and flight' to the 'rest-and-digest' mode, thus enhancing overall well-being.

The Perils of Chronic Stress

The modern world is a breeding ground for chronic stress. An overwhelming workload, the pressure of exams, social expectations and even unresolved emotional pain can all trigger a prolonged SNS response. Living with your 'foot on the gas' for extended periods takes a toll:

- **Fat Accumulation:** During SNS activation, the body shifts to fat storage mode, often leading to increased abdominal fat—a survival mechanism from our ancestors that assumes food scarcity in times of stress.
- **Reduced Fertility:** Reproductive functions take a back seat during stress; the body isn't interested in procreation when it feels threatened, leading to fertility issues for many chronically stressed individuals.
- **Mental Fatigue:** Constant SNS activity exhausts the mind, contributing to anxiety, mood swings and even depression.

Real-Life Scenarios of SNS–PNS Shifts

We all navigate these states daily:

- **Presentation at Work:** Before a crucial presentation, your SNS is in full swing—your heart races, your palms sweat and you're on high alert. After delivering it, taking deep breaths or engaging in a mindful walk can activate the PNS, bringing calm and clarity back.
- **Running into a Crisis:** You're driving when another car suddenly swerves into your lane. Your SNS jolts you into action, enabling you to react quickly. Once the danger has passed, sitting quietly and focusing on your breath will help you return to the restorative PNS state.
- **Exam Stress:** For students, exams represent a perceived threat. The SNS responds by creating anxiety, rapid heartbeats and heightened focus. After the exams, engaging in a fun, relaxing activity, like meeting friends or exercising, can shift the body back to a PNS state.

Exploring the Vagus Nerve: The Key to Relaxation

Central to the PNS's ability to restore balance is the vagus nerve, a cranial nerve that acts as the primary conduit between the brain and many vital organs, including the heart, lungs and digestive tract. This nerve plays a crucial role in regulating the body's rest-and-digest mode. When stimulated, it can lower the heart rate, decrease blood pressure and promote a profound sense of calm.

Techniques to Stimulate the Vagus Nerve

There are practical and accessible ways to stimulate the vagus nerve and promote relaxation:

- **Cold Exposure:** Splashing cold water on your face or even taking a cold shower can activate the vagus nerve, inducing a state of calm.
- **Humming or Chanting:** The vibrations produced by humming or chanting directly stimulate the vagus nerve, encouraging relaxation. This is why practices like chanting 'Om' in yoga or even singing softly can be so soothing.
- **Gargling:** Simple acts like gargling with water can stimulate the vagus nerve. Although it may seem unusual, it's a quick technique for activating the PNS.
- **Mindful Breath Work:** Slow, rhythmic breathing, especially with an emphasis on extended exhales, helps engage the vagus nerve and shift the body into a calm state.

These techniques demonstrate that even small, everyday actions can significantly influence the nervous system, helping us manage stress and promoting long-term health.

The following pages of the book explores these techniques in a lot more detail.

The Gut–Brain Connection: A Two-Way Street

The nervous system is not only about the brain and spinal cord. A growing body of research is uncovering the profound link between our gut health and our mental well-being—a connection known as the gut–brain axis. The gut, often referred to as our 'second brain', houses millions of neurons and is a vital player in the regulation of mood and stress.

How Stress Affects the Gut

When the SNS is overactive, blood is directed away from the digestive tract, causing a range of digestive issues. This is why stress can often lead to indigestion, irritable bowel syndrome (IBS) or other gut disturbances. The gut's health is intricately linked to our emotional state:

- **Gut Microbiome:** Chronic stress can negatively affect the balance of bacteria in our gut, known as the microbiome. An unhealthy microbiome can, in turn, influence our mood and anxiety levels, creating a vicious cycle.
- **Serotonin Production:** A significant portion of serotonin—the 'feel-good' hormone—is produced in the gut. When stress disrupts gut health, it can affect serotonin levels, leading to mood imbalances.

Conversely, a calm, well-regulated nervous system can enhance digestion, nutrient absorption and overall gut health, leading to better mental clarity and mood stability.

How to Create a Healthy Nervous System Balance

Our nervous system is a remarkable, finely tuned instrument that guides how we respond to life's challenges and joys. Achieving true well-being lies in finding a delicate balance—honouring the protective power of the SNS while nurturing the restorative, healing embrace of the PNS.

The goal is not to avoid SNS activation entirely, but to cultivate ways to spend more time in the PNS state. Our healing, recovery and overall resilience depend on our ability to step back from stress and find calm regularly.

In the following pages, you'll discover seventy-five science-backed strategies to encourage PNS activation. From deep breathing and mindful pauses to lighting a candle and spending time in nature, these simple, often overlooked practices can help you invite a sense of inner calm and balance. Cultivating these small but impactful habits can bring a shift towards greater harmony in your daily life.

We hope you'll find a few—or perhaps all—of these strategies that resonate with you and integrate them into your lifestyle. Remember, the key to true well-being isn't eliminating stress entirely but learning to navigate it with grace and resilience.

Part 2

75 Simple Ways of Moving from SNS to PNS

1

Cyclic Sigh/Physiological Sigh

If you've ever observed your breathing while crying or sobbing, you might notice a pattern of short, quick breaths followed by a long, audible sigh. This is the body's natural attempt to calm itself when overwhelmed with emotion. The *physiological sigh*, also known as the *cyclic sigh* is essentially a deliberate use of this mechanism, without the tears. When we use this technique consciously, we tap into a deeply ingrained calming process, designed to help us handle stress.

It is a breathing exercise rooted in nature and science. It taps into the body's innate mechanisms to shift from a state of nervous system dysregulation—marked by heightened stress, anxiety or panic—to a state of balance and calm.

It is a breathing pattern that involves two consecutive inhales followed by an extended exhale through the mouth. Here's a step-by-step guide to practising it:

First Inhale: Take a deep breath through your nose, filling your lungs.

Second Inhale: Without exhaling, take a smaller, quicker second breath, adding more air into the lungs.

Extended Exhale: Exhale slowly and completely through your mouth, with pursed lips, as if you're letting out a long sigh.

Repeating this cycle for six to seven times can bring about a sense of calm. The first inhale helps fill your lungs, while the second inhale is crucial for expanding the air sacs that might have collapsed, allowing for a deeper intake of oxygen. The slow, controlled exhale through pursed lips allows for a more complete release of carbon dioxide, which helps activate the PNS. This is what helps slow down the heart rate and brings about a soothing effect on the entire body.

The mechanism of the physiological sigh has been studied in recent years by neuroscientists like Dr Andrew Huberman, a professor at Stanford University. His research has shed light on how this practice works at a neurological level to help regulate the ANS. He and his team found that practising cyclic sighing increased participants' ability to manage stress effectively and improved overall well-being. The technique works by increasing the intake of oxygen and releasing carbon dioxide more effectively, which has a direct impact on reducing the physiological markers of stress, such as heart rate and blood pressure.

Another study, published in *Frontiers in Psychology*, explored the link between cyclic sighing and the PNS. It showed that the controlled exhalation phase of the sigh activates the vagus nerve, which plays a crucial role in managing the body's stress response. This activation leads to a slower heart rate and a decrease in the release of stress hormones, like cortisol, promoting a sense of calm and relaxation.

The physiological sigh is a powerful tool for managing anxiety and even panic attacks. During moments of intense stress, anxiety or a panic attack, our breathing often becomes rapid and shallow—a response known as *hyperventilation*. This kind of breathing can cause an imbalance between oxygen and carbon dioxide levels in the blood, leading to dizziness, increased heart rate and feelings of panic. The cyclic sigh counteracts this by emphasizing a deep and controlled exhale, which helps to restore the balance of gases in the bloodstream and prevent hyperventilation.

Here's why it works:

1. **Balances Oxygen and Carbon Dioxide Levels:** The second inhale in the cyclic sigh helps to open small

air sacs (alveoli) in the lungs, increasing oxygen intake. The long exhale helps release carbon dioxide, preventing the feeling of light-headedness and restoring equilibrium in the bloodstream.

2. **Activates the Vagus Nerve:** The vagus nerve is a major player in the PNS, which helps to calm the body. The extended exhalation during the cyclic sigh directly stimulates the vagus nerve, slowing down the heart rate and bringing a sense of relaxation.
3. **Shifts the Nervous System from Fight-or-Flight to Rest-and-Digest:** When stressed or anxious, the sympathetic nervous system (responsible for the fight-or-flight response) is often in overdrive. The cyclic sigh helps counterbalance this by promoting the activation of the PNS, which is key to relaxation. This shift can reduce feelings of panic and promote a sense of grounding and control.

Here's how one can use this breathing technique in their daily life:

- **Before a Stressful Event:** If you're about to give a presentation, take a few minutes to perform 6–7 cycles of the cyclic sigh. It can help to calm pre-event nerves, bringing you into a more focused and balanced state.
- **During a Panic Attack:** When you feel anxiety surging, stop and practise 6–7 cycles of the sigh. This helps to slow down rapid breathing and prevent the escalation of panic.
- **As a Daily Ritual:** Incorporating the physiological sigh into your morning or bedtime routine can have lasting benefits for managing stress throughout the day or unwinding in the evening.

So, whether you're seeking relief from daily stressors, need a tool to manage anxiety or simply want to feel more grounded, the *physiological sigh* can guide you back to calm, one breath at a time.

2

Wind Chimes

Have you ever found yourself enchanted by the gentle tinkling of wind chimes swaying in the breeze? Whether hanging from a balcony, gracing a front porch or adorning a garden, these delicate instruments have an undeniable ability to draw our attention and captivate our senses.

Wind chimes have a rich cultural history that dates back thousands of years. Their origins can be traced to ancient civilizations, including China, where they were first used as a form of protection and to summon spirits. Traditionally, Chinese wind chimes were made from metal and bamboo, often hung outside homes to ward off evil spirits and attract good fortune. Over time, their purpose evolved, and they became cherished decorative pieces, celebrated for their musical qualities and serene presence.

In Japan, wind chimes, known as *Furin*, are an integral part of summer culture. They are often made of glass and produce delicate, tinkling sounds that are thought to cool the senses on hot days. In both cultures, the enchanting sounds of wind chimes symbolize peace and tranquillity, aligning perfectly with their role in nervous system regulation.

The Science Behind Sound: How Wind Chimes Work

At the heart of the soothing effects of wind chimes lies the science of sound and its profound impact on our physiology.

Sound waves, produced by the vibrations of the chimes as they move in the wind, travel through the air and interact with our auditory system. This process engages our brain's auditory cortex, which processes sound and can trigger emotional responses.

The auditory system has direct connections to the limbic system, the part of the brain responsible for emotions and memory. This connection means that the sounds of wind chimes can evoke feelings of peace, nostalgia and comfort. Research has shown that certain sound frequencies can influence brainwave patterns, promoting relaxation and reducing stress. A study published in *Psychological Science* suggests that pleasant sounds, including music and natural sounds, can lower cortisol levels, a hormone associated with stress.

The gentle, melodious sounds produced by wind chimes engage the PNS. As the PNS activates, heart rate decreases, blood pressure lowers and the mind transitions from a state of alertness to relaxation.

Studies published on platforms like PubMed and National Center for Biotechnology Information (NCBI) have explored how exposure to soothing sounds, including those created by wind chimes, can induce relaxation and promote cardiovascular health.

1. **Impact on Blood Pressure and Heart Rate:** One study by Lee et al. (2017) examined the effects of sound therapy on patients with hypertension. The researchers found that participants who were exposed to calming sounds, including wind chimes, exhibited significant reductions in both systolic and diastolic blood pressure. The study concluded that sound therapy could serve as a complementary approach for managing hypertension, enhancing the effectiveness of traditional medical treatments.
2. **Stress Reduction and Heart Rate Variability:** Another significant study, published in *Frontiers in Psychology*,

analysed the effects of various soundscapes on individuals under stress. The findings indicated that exposure to natural sounds, including wind chimes, significantly increased heart rate variability (HRV)—a key indicator of PNS activity. Increased HRV is associated with a better ability to cope with stress and greater overall health.

3. **Brainwave Activity:** Research conducted by Thoma et al. (2013) demonstrated that sound frequencies, particularly those found in soothing music and natural sounds, can influence brainwave activity. Participants, who listened to calming sounds, showed a shift towards alpha and theta brainwaves, which are associated with relaxation and a meditative state.

To harness the calming effects of wind chimes, consider incorporating them into your daily environment. Here are a few suggestions:

1. **Choose the Right Chime:** Select wind chimes that resonate with you. The material, size and tone can greatly influence the sound. Bamboo chimes produce softer, warmer tones, while metal chimes create sharper, more resonant sounds.
2. **Placement Matters:** Hang wind chimes in areas where you spend significant time, such as your garden, balcony or near windows. This allows you to enjoy their soothing sounds throughout the day.
3. **Create a Relaxation Space:** Dedicate a corner of your home as a relaxation zone, complete with comfortable seating, plants and wind chimes. This space can serve as a retreat for meditation or quiet reflection.
4. **Mindful Listening:** Take a moment to sit quietly and listen to the chimes as they respond to the wind. Focus on their sound, letting it guide you into a state of mindfulness. This practice can be particularly effective in reducing anxiety and promoting emotional balance.

Wind chimes are more than mere decorations; they are powerful instruments that can help us restore balance in our lives. So, the next time you hear the gentle tinkling of wind chimes, take a moment to pause, breathe and allow their soothing sounds to carry you to a place of peace and harmony.

3

Go Slump Dump Pump

Think about this million-dollar question that plagues us all:

What is the root cause of unhappiness in our lives today?

- Stress?
- Anxiety?
- Fear?
- Insecurity?
- Comparison?
- Emotional baggage of the past?
- Resentment?
- Guilt?
- Hatred?
- Anger?
- Jealousy?
- The inability to forgive?

The list is almost never-ending, isn't it?

Yes, these emotions are part and parcel of life. However, the truth is that when they become chronic, they weigh us down. When you make them deep-seated, they manifest into symptoms and disease, over time. I am not the only one saying this. Medical science, research and common sense point to this intricate connection between our emotions and physical health.

When you harbour negative emotions within you, these start to eat you from the inside, creating a lower immune response, increasing inflammation and making you vulnerable to a host of diseases.

Many of us indeed live jet-set lives. We all have responsibilities. Sometimes, we become greedy and aspire for more than we can handle, and then our health problems start slowing us down. Some of us are in situations where our lives are difficult. Many people work two or three jobs to keep their families afloat, commute for 2 hours every day and, when they return home, they take care of the household chores, too, because there is no one to support them. Everyone's lives and struggles are different. We cannot judge others because we do not know what battles they are fighting.

That being said, amidst all these highs and lows, wins and losses, peaks and curveballs, no matter where we come from and what lives we live, there is one thing we all need. Relaxation. Sounds utopian, right? Only, it is not.

Truth bomb: Relaxation is not a choice. It is what the human body needs to survive and thrive.

You have the SNS and the PNS. While the SNS is responsible for your stress or flight/fight response, your PNS is where you rest, digest and regenerate—the state in which you grow, repair, digest your food and fall asleep.

Today, there are people talking about longevity and selling pills and supplements. I am not here to judge that. However, you must know this: **The more time you spend in the SNS, the faster you age.**

You could be popping all the expensive supplements and following the fifteen-step action plans that your longevity experts give you. **But the more stressed out you are, the faster you age.**

Is all stress bad? No. There are good and bad stressors. For instance, a cold shower or heat like a sauna or steam—these short-duration stressors can benefit you. However, what can you do when the frustration and angst of the day are weighing you down and cluttering your mind and it seems like there's no way out? I want to teach you a simple technique to relax instantly.

We have thousands of clients around the world who consult with us. Ninety per cent of them deal with jet-set lives and chronic stress. Mums out there with kids and work to handle, dads with issues, troubled young teenagers—everyone is stressed. People are in a hustle culture, where they think that doing more will get more results. I am here to empower you with this powerful technique. In the last few years, I have taught this to hundreds of my patients, and the results are exceptional.

All you need is 3–5 minutes to move into the PNS from the SNS.

S.D.P.: Slump, Dump and Pump

It's a technique that I came up with to create instant relaxation.

Where can you practise SDP? Wherever you are.

Step 1: Slump

You may be stressed, but did you know that you could still trick your body and mind?

All you need to do is find a comfortable position.

- Sit down in a chair or the couch. For the first time, I will ask you to do this—do not keep your back straight or sit erect.
- Just slump.
- Drop your head, in whatever direction is natural to you, and relax.
- Leave your hands be. They could be in your lap or dangling.
- Close your eyes.
- Once you have slumped, take a deep breath. A deep inhale.

- As you exhale, keep slumping more into a position of comfort. It could look odd, lazy, slouched—it doesn't matter.
- Follow every deep inhale with an exhale and slump further.

Picture a bag or a sack of potatoes. When you lift it, it is bulky, and the potatoes keep moving around. When you put it down, a couple of potatoes roll around in the sack and find a comfortable place to settle. It's called slumping.

If you have ever been in a hammock, you know it doesn't keep your back straight. Once you're in it, it takes the shape of your body. You relax with the sea around you. That is what slumping must feel like. You have completed Step 1.

Step 2: Dump

D stands for Dump. Not a literal dump, but a mental or mind dump.

- Think of it like this—every morning, we take a dump, or poop, to eliminate waste and toxins from the body.
- In the mind dump, we recollect everything that's happened in the last hour, day or since the hour you woke up.
- Think about anything negative that made you upset, angry or frustrated. It could be an event, a person or a thing.
- Now, visualize yourself dumping it out of your brain.
- Picture a trashcan and simply take out stuff from your mind and dump it in that trashcan—throwing out all that negativity or anything that didn't go well for you. That negative email, comment, heated debate on social media—just dump it out of your brain. I like to visualize a hand going into my head and dumping it into a trashcan.

You have now successfully slumped and taken a mind dump. Your mind is now empty. It is time to pump.

Step 3: Pump

In the pump phase, create a space for conductive and empowering thoughts to enter.

- Pump positive thoughts and instances into your mind—the ones that make you feel warm and happy; something or someone you are grateful for. Think about things that make you happy, what you are grateful for and what excites you. Pump in its goodness.
- Visualize the people you love—your parents, siblings, child or partner, recall a comment or a gesture that moved you. Pump it into your mind.
- It doesn't matter how big or small the thought is. If nothing comes to mind, just count the small blessings.
- Embrace this feeling. You might want to stay here longer because it feels so good.
- With that, you have reached the end of Step 3. You have successfully dumped and pumped.

It may sound complicated at first, but it isn't. We have been doing this with our clients, and the number of testimonials that have been floating around proves its power.

The other day, someone wrote to me, *'Luke, after I finished the S.D.P. exercise, my mind just feels lighter through the day.'*

How is this different from meditation? One of the differences is that you do not need to silence your mind or thoughts.

If you have more negative thoughts, let the dumping process be longer. The goal is to pump your mind back with good thoughts.

Some may wonder, *'What if there is nothing to dump? What if I have had a good day?'* Then, move straight to the pump phase and relax.

We teach it to our patients undergoing chemotherapy sitting in the hospital. We reach them to slump and dump all the negativity that's going on in their minds as the chemo goes in, to pump in thoughts of what they want.

Many clients who tried this before hitting the hay say, *'Luke, we are sleeping like babies.'*

It is simple. You dump the negative and pump the positive. The simple act moves you from the SNS into the PNS. This is the system where you want to spend most of your day and life in. It equals longevity, immunity, low inflammation, repair, cell growth, human growth hormone, inner peace, relaxation and more.

Three to 5 minutes is all it takes. The next time thoughts and situations pull you down, excuse yourself and do a **slump–dump–pump.** Try it today.

4

Listening to Birdsongs

Nature has a remarkable ability to soothe frazzled nerves. Birdsong serves as a marker of safety in nature, as birds typically sing in the absence of danger. Their songs are often most prominent during dawn and dusk, times when predators are less active. When birds sing, it is an indication that their immediate environment is safe, allowing them to engage in social communication, attract mates and establish territories. The presence of songbirds signals to other creatures, including humans, that it is a moment of safety in the ecosystem.

Several experiments and studies have been conducted to explore the impact of birdsong on human psychological and physiological responses. A study published in *Scientific Reports,* by Aletta Bonnema and colleagues, examined how exposure to different soundscapes, including natural environments with birdsongs, affected stress levels. Participants who listened to natural sounds reported significantly lower levels of stress and anxiety compared to those exposed to urban noise. This study suggests that birdsongs can help create a calming atmosphere that promotes relaxation.

Another research, conducted at the University of Exeter, investigated how exposure to birdsongs affects cognitive performance and mood. The study found that participants who listened to recordings of birdsongs while completing tasks, demonstrated improved focus and cognitive functioning compared to those in a silent environment or exposed to urban sounds. This enhancement in cognitive performance highlights the benefits of natural soundscapes for mental clarity and well-being.

A study published in *Frontiers in Psychology* explored the physiological effects of listening to natural sounds, including birdsongs. The researchers measured participants' heart rates and cortisol levels while they listened to various soundscapes. Results indicated that natural sounds significantly lowered heart rates and cortisol levels, which are markers of stress. Birdsongs were particularly effective in promoting relaxation and reducing physiological stress responses.

In a study published in *Environmental Research*, researchers examined the effects of nature sounds on recovery from stress. Participants were placed in a controlled environment and exposed to either urban noise or recordings of natural sounds, including birdsongs. Those who listened to birdsongs reported feeling calmer and more relaxed, and their physiological stress markers showed a significant improvement. This research reinforces the idea that birdsongs can facilitate recovery from stressful situations.

A study conducted by researchers at the University of Sussex investigated the psychological effects of listening to birdsongs. The participants, who listened to birdsongs for a brief period, reported enhanced mood and a reduction in feelings of anxiety. This finding suggests that birdsongs can act as a natural antidote to the stressors of modern life, promoting emotional well-being.

The Connection to Human Experience

1. **Psychological Safety and Auditory Cues**
   In a study published in *Environmental Research*, researchers examined the effects of nature sounds on recovery from stress. Participants were placed in a controlled environment and exposed to either urban noise or recordings of natural sounds, including

birdsongs. Birdsong serves as an auditory cue that communicates safety to us. In the same way that birds sing to assert their presence, humans may subconsciously interpret these sounds as signals that the environment is safe. This can lead to a reduction in anxiety and stress, facilitating a more balanced state of mind.

2. **Mindfulness and Connection to Nature**
   The practice of mindfulness—being present in the moment—can be greatly enhanced by immersing ourselves in natural soundscapes. A study conducted by the University of Exeter found that spending time in nature, particularly listening to birdsongs, significantly improved participants' mood and reduced anxiety.
3. **Soundscapes and Stress Recovery**
   The calming effects of birdsongs can also promote recovery from stress. A study published in *Environmental Research* found that individuals exposed to soundscapes, featuring birdsongs, showed lower physiological markers of stress, such as heart rate and blood pressure. These findings suggest that birdsongs create a nurturing sound environment that can help restore balance to our nervous system.

To make the most of the calming effects of bird songs, here's what you can do:

1. Engaging in activities such as birdwatching or simply sitting in a park and listening to birdsongs can immerse you in the calming rhythms of nature.
2. Incorporate mindful listening into your routine. Find a quiet space to close your eyes and listen to recordings of birdsongs or, ideally, experience them live, in nature.
3. If access to natural environments is limited, consider creating a sound sanctuary at home. Use recordings

of birdsongs to fill your space, particularly during moments of stress or when you need to unwind. The gentle sounds of birds can mimic the safety cues found in nature.

Just as birds thrive in moments of calm, we, too, can benefit from the serene messages conveyed through their songs.

5

Embracing Imperfections

Imagine standing before a mirror, scrutinizing every detail of your reflection. The blemish on your cheek, the stray hair out of place, the slight crease in your clothes—each flaw feels magnified. Now, take a moment to ask yourself: How does this relentless need for perfection affect your daily life?

Perfectionism isn't just a quirky trait; it's a psychological construct that has been extensively studied. Research published in the *Journal of Personality* reveals that perfectionists often set unrealistically high standards for themselves, which can lead to chronic dissatisfaction, anxiety and even depression (Visvalingam et al., 2023). A study published in *Contemporary Family Therapy* found that individuals with perfectionistic tendencies are more likely to experience burnout and emotional distress (Holden and Jeanfreau, 2023).

When we chase an ideal that is inherently unattainable, we set ourselves up for failure. Perfectionism thrives on comparison, often leading us to feel inadequate when we inevitably fall short. Yet, beneath this drive for flawlessness lies a fear of judgement and rejection. Understanding this connection is the first step towards letting go.

Begin by recognizing this: Perfection is a lie we're often sold.

The media and movies frequently portray flawless relationships, ideal lives and flawless appearances, leading people to believe that perfection is attainable. Many of us spend excessive amounts of time, money and energy trying to reach impossible standards, yet perfection remains forever out of reach.

Why? Because change is constant and inevitable, whether it is people, relationships and circumstances. When we embrace imperfection in ourselves and others, we open the door to compassion and understanding. Instead of striving for perfection, aim for excellence. Focus on growing your skills and improving yourself in meaningful ways. Let go of the need for external validation because you don't need everyone to agree with or like you.

The world is not perfect; it's a complex mix of challenges, beauty and flaws. Most perfectionists often experience irritability and anger because their high expectations are rarely met. The world will never be exactly as they envision it. Don't let these curated images on social media fool you into believing perfection exists. This unquenchable need for perfection can affect you in more ways than you imagine.

The Negative Impact of Perfectionism

Many perfectionists struggle to accept flaws in their partners, children or friends. This can lead to conflicts and tension. For some, aiming for perfection is often tied to an inflated ego and pride, making it hard to accept constructive criticism or to learn from mistakes.

In relationships, people often enter with unrealistic expectations, seeking a 'perfect' partner. However, as individuals and relationships evolve, these expectations become impossible to sustain. The constant demand for perfection leads to disappointment, resentment and conflict. A person fixated on having the 'perfect' partner may find themselves critiquing flaws or feeling dissatisfied, even in a healthy relationship.

In parenting, striving to be the 'perfect' parent often means setting unrealistic expectations for children's behaviour, achievements or development. When children naturally fall short, it creates frustration for both the parent and child. This pressure strains the parent–child relationship and stifles the child's emotional growth, making it harder for them to develop resilience and self-acceptance.

In the workplace, the pursuit of perfection can be detrimental. People may invest excessive time in tasks, overlooking their well-being and personal relationships to produce flawless work. This often leads to burnout, decreased productivity and strained connections with colleagues. For instance, someone preparing a 'perfect' presentation may spend all night refining it, sacrificing sleep and personal time, only to feel dissatisfied with the outcome in the morning.

This creates an everyday cycle of dissatisfaction and overshadows your life's most simple pleasures.

The Power of Imperfections

What if we shifted our perspective and embraced our imperfections? Research from the University of California published in the *Personality and Social Psychology Bulletin* suggests that individuals who accept their flaws are more likely to experience higher levels of self-compassion and a deeper connection with themselves and others (Zhang, Chen, and Tomova Shakur, 2020).

I want you to illustrate this with *Kintsugi* and *Wabi-Sabi*—two beautiful Japanese concepts that celebrate imperfection and transience.

Kintsugi, which translates to 'golden joinery', is the practice of repairing broken pottery with lacquer, dusted or mixed with powdered gold, silver or platinum. Instead of hiding the cracks and imperfections, Kintsugi highlights them, creating a piece of art that is unique and full of history. This technique not only restores functionality, but also transforms the object into something even more beautiful than the original.

Kintsugi embodies the idea that breakage and repair are part of the life cycle. Just as a broken pot can become a work of art, our own experiences—both joyful and painful—shape who we are. It teaches us to view our scars and imperfections as valuable elements of our personal narrative, rather than as something to be ashamed of.

Wabi-Sabi is a broader aesthetic and philosophical concept that celebrates the beauty of the imperfect, impermanent and incomplete. It encourages us to appreciate the transient nature of life, recognizing that nothing lasts forever and that beauty can be found in the simplest of things.

It hinges on three principles:

- **Impermanence:** Acknowledging that everything is in a state of flux and that change is natural.
- **Imperfection:** Embracing flaws and irregularities, finding beauty in the asymmetrical and the incomplete.
- **Simplicity:** Valuing minimalism and the unadorned, focusing on authenticity over ostentation.

Wabi-Sabi invites us to slow down and appreciate the moment, find joy in the mundane and recognize that our imperfections—both physical and emotional—are what make us uniquely human.

In a world that often pressures us to present a polished exterior, embracing Kintsugi and Wabi-Sabi allows us to find peace and beauty in our authentic selves.

Your Journey to Embracing Imperfection

What can you do to embrace your imperfections? Here are some simple exercises to get you started.

- **Reflect on Your Perfectionism:** Start by identifying the areas of your life where perfectionism shows up. Is it in your work, relationships or appearance? Write down specific instances where you felt compelled to achieve an unattainable standard. Reflect on how these experiences made you feel.

Exercise: Create a 'Perfectionism Inventory' list. Write down three situations where your desire for perfection held you back, and next to each, jot down how you could have embraced imperfection instead.

- **Reframe Your Self-Talk:** Perfectionism often breeds negative self-talk. Challenge these thoughts by reframing them. For example, instead of saying, 'I can't fail,' try, 'I can learn from my mistakes.'

  Exercise: Each morning, write down a positive affirmation that counters your perfectionist tendencies. Repeat it throughout the day. For example, 'I am enough just as I am.'
- **Practice Self-Compassion:** Embracing imperfection requires a compassionate approach towards yourself. Understand that making mistakes is part of being human.

  Exercise: When you encounter a mistake, write a compassionate letter to yourself as if you were speaking to a friend. Acknowledge your feelings and offer encouragement and understanding.
- **Engage in Creative Exploration:** Allow yourself to be imperfect in a creative way. Engage in an activity that you enjoy but don't feel the need to excel at. Whether it's painting, dancing or cooking, let go of the pressure to achieve a perfect result.

  Exercise: Set a timer for 20 minutes and create something—anything! Allow yourself to make 'mistakes' and notice how liberating it feels. I tried this on my work trip to Switzerland's Clinic Le Alpes, where art therapy is used for those trying to overcome addiction. What a beautiful experience it was just to let the paint cover the canvas with its own flow.
- **Celebrate Your Flaws:** Take time to acknowledge and celebrate your unique qualities and quirks. Consider how these imperfections contribute to your character and individuality.

Exercise: Create a 'Flaw Celebration' jar. Write down three of your perceived flaws and how they make you uniquely you. Whenever you feel overwhelmed by perfectionism, read these notes.

Remember, embracing imperfection is not about giving up your ambitions or settling for mediocrity. It's about finding freedom in your flaws and recognizing that they contribute to your unique narrative.

Think back to the last time you felt connected to someone—wasn't it often during a moment of vulnerability? Those raw, unfiltered exchanges foster deeper bonds and create a sense of belonging. By embracing your imperfections, you allow others to do the same.

In a world that often values perfection, choosing to embrace your flaws is an act of courage and authenticity. Remind yourself every once in a while, that you are enough, exactly as you are.

6

Lighting a Candle

Have you ever wondered why you feel so calm and relaxed when you walk into a space lit by candles? Or, why are candle-lit dinners considered the epitome of romance? Why do hotels and spas use these flickering flames to create an atmosphere of pure relaxation? There's more to it than just ambiance—it's science!

Candles, campfires and bonfires emit a soft, warm light that includes infrared radiation, which can help activate the PNS. It is the state where true relaxation can occur. This is why candles in your bedroom can be transformative. Of course, the right placement and safety measures matter. But not just any candle will do. Quality matters, too.

Source natural or purely organic candles to avoid inhaling the harmful chemicals found in low-quality scented candles.

So, why not start a new evening ritual? Collect a few beautiful candles and light them as you wind down in the evening. It is especially effective for those struggling with sleep issues.

The gentle flicker of candlelight mimics the natural rhythms of firelight, which humans have evolved to associate with safety, warmth and community. Unlike harsh, artificial lighting, this soft, moving light causes less strain on our eyes and can help signal to our brains that it is time to unwind, making it easier to relax or fall asleep.

Personally, I am a candle lover. I have them in nearly every corner of my home, and the difference they make is incredible. The energy shift, the connection to nature and the soothing power of natural light are remarkable.

Many candles are infused with essential oils or natural scents that can further enhance relaxation. For example, lavender is known for its calming properties, while eucalyptus can promote clear breathing and mental clarity. The olfactory system (our sense of smell) is closely linked to the limbic system in the brain, which governs emotions and memory, so certain scents can trigger feelings of comfort and well-being.

Candles make us feel good because they engage in multiple senses—sight, smell and touch—in ways that naturally promote relaxation, comfort and mindfulness.

Lighting a candle can be a mindful act, a simple ritual that helps us slow down and become present. The act of striking a match, watching the flame catch and observing the candle burn can help us focus on the moment, reducing anxiety and promoting a sense of peace.

Pro tip: If you want to take this simple practice of lighting a candle even further, light it and stare at the flame. Try not to blink for as long as you can. The practice finds its root in ancient yoga and is known as ***Trataka***. It will declutter your mind, clear your tear ducts and enhance focus and concentration.

Have Candlelight Dinners

There's something almost magical about a candlelight dinner. Whether it's a carefully planned date night or a spontaneous decision to light a candle during a weekday dinner, the soft glow of candlelight can transform an ordinary meal into a moment of serenity. It is such a gentle ritual for down-regulating the nervous system. However, beyond its romantic reputation, candlelight can have a powerful calming effect on our nervous system.

Studies in psychology and neuroscience reveal that our nervous system responds favourably to soft, warm lighting, like the gentle flicker of a candle. It supports the activation of the PNS.

A study published in *Chronobiology International* highlighted that exposure to dim light during evening hours can support melatonin production, the hormone responsible for regulating sleep cycles (Tähkämö, Partonen, and Pesonen, 2018). In other words, the soothing atmosphere of a candlelight dinner can make it easier to unwind, digest and even prepare for a restful night's sleep.

Why Candlelight Dinners Feel Special

Beyond the scientific evidence, there's a unique charm that comes with dining by candlelight. It's not just the warm, ambient glow—it's the experience that it creates. The slow, rhythmic flicker of a candle invites a sense of presence, helping us stay anchored in the moment. It encourages slower eating, richer conversations and a deeper connection with our surroundings. The visual appeal of a candlelit table is also worth noting. The softened glow adds depth and dimension, making even a simple dinner look and feel more beautiful. This environment plays into what psychologists call the 'aesthetic experience'—the sense of pleasure we derive from visual harmony.

Studies in the *Journal of Environmental Psychology* suggest that people feel greater positive emotions in aesthetically pleasing environments, which can translate into better mood and reduced stress levels (González-Espinar et al., 2023). This is, perhaps, why candlelight has been used in rituals and celebrations across cultures for centuries—it elevates the ordinary, transforming it into something special.

The beauty of a candlelight dinner is that it doesn't need to be elaborate. You don't have to reserve it for anniversaries or special occasions. Sometimes, a candle on your dining table, during a typical weekday dinner, is enough to enhance the atmosphere. It's a simple way to break from routine and make the mundane feel meaningful. By turning off bright lights and lighting a candle, you can create a pocket of calm in your day—a little ritual that invites relaxation into the moment.

Imagine coming home after a long day, the world still buzzing in your mind. The dinner table is set, and instead of reaching for the usual overhead lights, you light a candle. The warm glow slowly fills the room, and the day's stress seems to soften. You may find that you savour your meal more, taste the flavours more fully and engage in conversation more deeply. It's a practice that can bring mindfulness to the dinner table, helping you reconnect with yourself or your loved ones after the day's hustle.

Incorporating candlelight into your evening meals can be a gentle signal to your brain that the day's challenges are over, and it's time to transition into rest and recovery. It's a way to signal to your body that it's safe and that there's no need for vigilance, allowing your PNS to take charge.

Sometimes, it's the simplest of changes that make the biggest difference. So, the next time you find yourself overwhelmed or stressed, try lighting a candle at dinner and see how it transforms your evening. You might just discover a new favourite way to unwind.

7

Chanting/Humming

Humming and chanting are among the timeless practices that are rooted in ancient wisdom and backed by science. One of the most fascinating aspects of chanting and humming lies in the science of how sound vibrations impact the body's systems, especially the nervous system. When we chant or hum, we create vibrations within our body that stimulate the vagus nerve, promoting relaxation. These vibrations are particularly noticeable in the chest, throat and head, creating a resonance that stimulates the nerve. Studies published on PubMed and NCBI confirm that vagal stimulation, such as that which occurs during humming or chanting, has a calming effect on the nervous system, effectively slowing down heart rate and lowering blood pressure.

When humming or chanting, we sustain a single tone, which not only allows the mind to focus but also helps in 'switching off' external distractions. This steady, intentional sound brings the body back to a balanced state, much like the calming effect of a lullaby on a baby. The effect is immediate; a few minutes of focused humming can shift our physiological state from anxious and reactive to calm and centred.

Studies on Humming and Chanting

- **The Om Effect:** A study published on PubMed demonstrated that chanting 'Om' had significant effects on the limbic system, the emotional centre of the brain, leading to a reduction in stress and improvement in emotional resilience. Participants who practised Om chanting regularly reported reduced levels of anxiety and enhanced mood stability. Researchers suggest that the sound 'Om' stimulates the vagus nerve, which can improve both physical and mental health by promoting relaxation and emotional stability.

- ***Bhramari Pranayama* (Bee Humming):** Bhramari pranayama, also known as bee humming breath, has been shown to be effective in reducing blood pressure and heart rate. A study published by the *Journal of Alternative and Complementary Medicine* highlighted that regular practice of Bhramari breath reduces cortisol levels—the stress hormone—thereby reducing overall stress and promoting a sense of calm. This technique, commonly taught by yoga therapists, involves closing the eyes, taking a deep breath and humming on the exhale, creating a soothing vibration in the head and chest that promotes relaxation.
- **The Calming Power of Simple Humming:** Another study examined the effects of gentle, continuous humming, finding that it stimulated the production of nitric oxide, a molecule that improves blood flow and oxygen delivery throughout the body. Improved blood flow can help reduce tension in the body and promote a sense of relaxation, with positive effects on mood, immunity and even sleep quality.

Ways to Practise Chanting and Humming

These simple techniques can be practised anywhere, anytime, and they don't require much time or effort. Here are three methods to incorporate chanting and humming into your routine:

1. *Omkar* Chanting

Chanting 'Om' is said to represent the sound of the universe, the original vibration. In this practice, take a deep breath and chant a long, steady 'Om', feeling the resonance throughout your body. Focus on the vibration as it travels from your chest to your throat and head. Even a few minutes can produce profound relaxation effects, as it naturally stimulates the vagus nerve and helps activate the parasympathetic response.

2. Bee Humming (Bhramari Pranayama)

Practised widely in yoga, bee humming involves sitting comfortably, closing your eyes and taking a deep breath. Then, on the exhale, hum like a bee with your lips gently closed, feeling the 'mmmm' sound vibrate in your head and face. This sound produces a sensation that is incredibly soothing for the nervous system, helping to relieve tension and promote a deep state of relaxation.

3. Soft Humming

A soft, gentle hum, even with no particular tune, can be just as effective. Choose a pitch that feels comfortable, and hum softly, paying attention to the vibrations in your chest and throat. This quiet practice can be grounding and calming, offering a simple way to reset during a busy day. It's especially useful for those moments when you feel overwhelmed; a few deep breaths with soft humming can quickly bring you back to a calm state.

Dr Herbert Benson from Harvard Medical School, renowned for his work on the relaxation response, found that repetitive practices like chanting trigger the body's natural relaxation response. According to Dr Benson, any repetitive sound, including chanting or humming, can induce a meditative state, lower stress and improve focus.

These practices are simple, requiring no equipment or elaborate set-up, making them accessible to anyone. In a few mindful breaths, you can shift from a state of tension to one of calm, from 'fight-or-flight' to 'rest-and-digest'. So, the next time the world feels overwhelming, take a deep breath and let the sound of your own voice guide you back to balance.

8

Cold/Hot Therapy

Hot and cold therapy is not just a trend; it's a time-tested practice with roots in ancient traditions like Finnish saunas, Roman baths and cold water plunges. This form of therapy has gained recognition in the modern wellness world for its ability to affect the nervous system deeply, helping us shift from a state of stress to one of relaxation. Today, scientific research has explored and confirmed many of the benefits of alternating between hot and cold treatments, revealing how these therapies can help down-regulate an overactive nervous system.

The Science of Hot Therapy: Sauna and Steam

Hot therapy, through methods like saunas and steam baths, is known for promoting relaxation and reducing stress. Saunas, particularly popular in Nordic countries, involve sitting in a small room, heated to temperatures ranging between 70°C (158°F) and 100°C (212°F). This heat exposure raises the body's core temperature, inducing a state of deep relaxation.

A study published on PubMed explored the effects of sauna bathing on the ANS, showing that regular sauna use increases parasympathetic activity. The heat exposure causes blood vessels to dilate, improving circulation and creating a sense of calmness. At the same time, it promotes the release of endorphins, the body's natural 'feel-good' chemicals, which contribute to a sensation of well-being and reduced stress levels.

Steam baths offer similar benefits but include the added element of humidity. A steam bath typically operates at lower temperatures but with higher humidity levels, making it feel hotter. This combination can help to soothe muscles, ease respiratory conditions and create an environment conducive to deep relaxation. Steam therapy has been shown to support vagal tone, which is crucial for maintaining balance in the ANS. A well-regulated vagus nerve is associated with improved mood and better resilience to stress, as shown in research from NCBI.

The Role of Cold Therapy: Cold Showers and Plunges

Cold therapy, such as cold showers, plunges or ice baths, may seem intimidating at first, but its benefits to the nervous system are well-documented. When the body is exposed to cold, it triggers a physiological response known as 'cold-induced vasoconstriction', where blood vessels constrict to preserve core body heat. This process not only enhances circulation but also stimulates the vagus nerve, which plays a pivotal role in calming the body's stress response.

A study published on PubMed found that cold water immersion significantly activates the PNS, leading to a decrease in cortisol levels. The research showed that regular exposure to cold water helps increase the body's resilience to stress over time, making it easier to transition from a 'fight-or-flight' state to a state of relaxation.

Cold therapy has also been associated with a surge in norepinephrine, a neurotransmitter that plays a role in mood regulation and focus, making it beneficial not just for physical recovery but for mental well-being as well.

The Interplay between Hot and Cold: Contrast Therapy

Combining hot and cold therapy, often referred to as contrast therapy, can be particularly effective for balancing the nervous system. This technique involves alternating between hot and cold environments, such as moving from a sauna to a cold plunge or alternating between hot and cold showers. The contrast between the two temperatures creates a pumping effect in the blood vessels, which supports circulation, muscle recovery and overall relaxation.

Research in *Wounds International* highlights that contrast therapy can help lower inflammation in the body, making it a popular choice for athletes as well as individuals seeking stress relief. It's thought that this form of thermal cycling helps to 'reset' the ANS, providing a unique way to quickly shift from a state of tension to relaxation. The process of enduring both extremes encourages the body to adapt, leading to improved resilience against daily stressors.

Other Ancient and Traditional Bathing Practices

Throughout history, various cultures have embraced the benefits of hot and cold therapy through ancient bathing practices that combine these elements.

Hamams, or Turkish baths, offer a unique blend of heat and steam, allowing individuals to relax and cleanse themselves, both physically and mentally. These baths often include a sequence of experiences, starting with a warm room to open the pores, followed by a vigorous scrub and concluding with a cool rinse. This practice promotes relaxation and revitalization, enhancing overall well-being.

Roman baths were famous for their elaborate thermal bathing systems, often comprising hot, warm and cold pools. The ancient Romans believed in the therapeutic benefits of water, and their bathhouses were social centres, where people would gather to relax, socialize and rejuvenate. The use of alternating temperatures in these baths is a precursor to modern contrast therapy, emphasizing the timeless wisdom of utilizing heat and cold for health benefits.

Salt baths are another ancient tradition that integrates the healing properties of salt with temperature therapy. Salt is known for its detoxifying properties, and soaking in warm salt water can help alleviate muscle tension, improve skin health and promote relaxation. Modern wellness centres often offer salt therapy experiences, where individuals can enjoy the soothing benefits of salt, combined with heat.

In Japan, the practice of *onsen* (hot springs) provides another example of how ancient cultures utilized hot and cold therapies for relaxation and healing. Onsen bathing involves soaking in naturally heated, mineral-rich waters, often surrounded by serene nature. This practice not only aids in relaxation but also offers various health benefits, including improved circulation and skin rejuvenation.

The Positive Stress Response: Hormesis and Immune Boosting

Engaging in hot and cold therapy also taps into the concept of **hormesis**—the idea that exposure to low levels of stress can be beneficial to health. This mild stress prompts the body to adapt, leading to improved resilience and function.

Scientific studies have shown that both heat and cold exposure stimulate the production of protective proteins, particularly **heat shock proteins (HSPs)**. HSPs play a vital role in cellular protection, helping to prevent damage from stressors and promoting recovery. Research published by the NCBI indicates that HSPs help to mitigate inflammation, support immune function and enhance overall cellular health.

Additionally, regular exposure to controlled stressors, such as heat and cold, can strengthen the immune system, making the body more adept at handling various stressors.

For instance, a study published in the *Journal of Human Kinetics* found that regular sauna use can enhance immune response by increasing the production of white blood cells, which are essential for fighting infections.

Practical Application: Incorporating Hot and Cold Therapy into Daily Life

Integrating hot and cold therapy into your routine doesn't have to be complicated. Here are some simple practices you can try:

1. **Start with Saunas:** If you have access to a sauna (mostly in hotels or gym centres), try incorporating a session a few times every week. Aim for 15–30 minutes to experience the full benefits.
2. **Cold Showers:** Gradually introduce cold showers into your routine. Start with warm water and switch to cold for the last 30 seconds to a minute. Over time, you can increase the duration of cold exposure.
3. **Contrast Showers:** Alternate between hot and cold water in the shower. Start with warm water for a few minutes, then switch to cold for 30 seconds, and repeat several times.
4. **Embrace Ice Baths:** If you're adventurous, consider incorporating ice baths after intense workouts. Ensure that you gradually acclimatize your body to the cold.
5. **Warm Baths with Additives:** Create a calming bath experience at home by adding Epsom salts or essential oils like lavender.
6. **Explore Traditional Bathhouses:** If possible, visit local hamams or spas that offer ancient bathing practices to experience the benefits of hot and cold therapy in a traditional setting.

9

Massage

Imagine feeling your shoulders drop, your mind quieten down and the world around you fading into the background. That's the magic of a good massage. I've made it a priority to invest in wellness massages regularly. During my travels, I've had the privilege of experiencing some of the best massages, crafted by skilled experts who truly know how to work wonders on the body.

Beyond just the soothing touch, massages have a remarkable ability to help shift our bodies from SNS to PNS.

When you get a massage, your body's response is almost immediate. The gentle pressure, rhythmic movements and nurturing touch signal to your brain that it's safe to relax. Your heart rate slows down, your muscles unwind and your breathing becomes deeper and more rhythmic. It's like hitting the reset button for your entire system.

Traditional Massage Techniques from Around the World

Have you noticed how essential massages are for athletes' recovery, not only for relaxing muscles but also for optimizing physical performance, reducing injury risks and supporting overall well-being? After rigorous training sessions, muscle fibres can become tight, fatigued and susceptible to injury. Massages aid in releasing muscle tension, boosting circulation and promoting the body's natural healing processes, which can accelerate recovery time.

Indian Ayurvedic Massage *(Abhyanga)*

In Ayurveda, the ancient Indian healing system, Abhyanga, is a warm oil massage designed to balance the body's *doshas* (energies) and promote overall well-being. The use of herbal oils in Abhyanga improves circulation, reduces inflammation and has a grounding effect on the nervous system.

Thai Massage

This involves stretching, pressing and pulling movements along the body's energy lines. Practised widely across Thailand, this technique incorporates yoga-like stretches and pressure points to improve flexibility, increase joint mobility and stimulate the body's energy flow—making it ideal for athletes seeking increased flexibility and reduced stiffness.

Swedish Massage

Known for its long, flowing strokes and kneading, Swedish massage is a Western favourite for relaxation and rejuvenation.

Shiatsu (Japanese Massage)

Shiatsu, meaning 'finger pressure' in Japanese, uses targeted pressure along the body's meridians (energy pathways) to relieve pain, reduce tension and restore balance. For athletes, Shiatsu can help release tension in specific areas, promoting relaxation and flexibility essential for peak performance.

Lomi Lomi (Hawaiian Massage)

Originating from Hawaii, Lomi Lomi uses rhythmic, wave-like strokes that resemble the flow of water. This technique helps in releasing tension, promoting relaxation and balancing energy. It's gentle, yet deeply relaxing, for those who want a mild but effective recovery massage.

Kalari Chikitsa (Kalaripayattu Massage)

Originating in Kerala, Kalari Chikitsa is a unique form of massage associated with Kalaripayattu, one of the oldest martial arts. This technique uses herbal oils and focuses on specific *marma* points (energy centres) to improve flexibility, strength and endurance.

Traditional Baby Massages in India: A Nostalgic Ritual for Strength

In India, the tradition of massaging infants is a beloved ritual passed down through generations. Grandmothers or other older family members, usually take on this task with loving expertise, using gentle, rhythmic strokes and warm oil, often sesame or coconut, to build the baby's strength.

The massage helps in:

- Developing muscle tone
- Strengthening bones
- Enhancing flexibility
- Supporting physical milestones like crawling and walking
- Promoting better circulation
- Aiding digestion, relieving gas and reducing colic symptoms by stimulating bowel movements
- Relaxing them and making it easier for them to settle into deeper, more restful sleep
- Making them aware of their bodies, supporting coordination and motor skills for sensory development and self-soothing

This ritual is a bonding experience, filled with lullabies, gentle cooing and age-old stories.

If a gentle massage (in most cases, unless your doctor has advised you against it) can help a baby, it can certainly help you. Give yourself a break every now and then and book yourself a good massage. See if you sleep as soundly as a baby does!

Scientific Evidence Supporting Massage Therapy

- A study published in the *International Journal of Neuroscience* found that massage therapy reduced cortisol levels by up to 31 per cent, while increasing serotonin and dopamine by 28 per cent and 31 per cent, respectively (Field et al., 2005).
- Another study in *Biological Research for Nursing* revealed that participants who received regular massages showed significant reductions in both measures, suggesting that massage helps the body move into a more restful state (Olney, 2005). The rhythmic touch and pressure applied during a massage stimulate the vagus nerve—a major component of the PNS—which plays a key role in lowering heart rate, promoting digestion and enhancing relaxation.
- Research published in *the Journal of Alternative and Complementary Medicine* showed that massage therapy could improve the variability of heart rate, an indicator of a healthy PNS response (Kaye et al., 2008). Higher HRV is associated with better stress resilience, improved emotional regulation and overall cardiovascular health. This study concluded that massage therapy could be an effective non-invasive approach to managing stress and improving overall autonomic function.

Making the Most of Your Massage Experiences

1. Before you get a massage, take a moment to set an intention. It could be as simple as *'I allow myself to relax'* or *'I am here to let go.'* This mindset shift can make your massage even more effective.

2. As your massage begins, focus on your breath. Slow, deep breaths signal to your body that it's okay to relax and make it easier to shift into the PNS.
3. Different massages have different effects. A gentle Swedish massage is great for relaxation, while a deep-tissue massage might help release stubborn tension. Listen to your body and choose what feels right.
4. It's easy to let your mind wander but try to stay present with the sensations of the massage. Notice how each stroke feels and how your body responds. This mindfulness can deepen your relaxation.
5. Be adequately hydrated afterwards to help flush out toxins released during the massage.
6. Don't rush back into your day. Take a few extra minutes to sit quietly, feel all your feelings or just enjoy the afterglow of relaxation.

Massages are more than just a luxury—they're a beautiful way to reconnect with your body, release stress and remind yourself of the importance of rest. Don't wait till you find yourself overwhelmed. Allow yourself to unwind, one soothing touch at a time. Self-care is the best form of care.

10

Pets

Imagine returning home after a long, stressful day. Your mind races with the pressures of work, relationships and daily responsibilities. You step through the door, and there, waiting for you with a wagging tail or a gentle purr, is your pet. In that moment, the worries of the world seem to fade away. This simple, yet meaningful, interaction is not just a moment of joy; it is a powerful biological response that can help regulate the nervous system, thereby transitioning us from a state of stress to one of calm.

The human-animal bond is more than just companionship; it is a biological and psychological phenomenon that influences our emotional and physiological states. When we interact with pets, several scientific mechanisms come into play that can help shift our nervous system from sympathetic dominance to parasympathetic activity. Research has demonstrated that petting animals leads to the release of oxytocin, a hormone associated with bonding, love and social connection. In a study published in *Science*, researchers found that oxytocin levels increased significantly after individuals interacted with dogs, promoting feelings of affection and connection (Odendaal and Meintjes, 2003).

Furthermore, oxytocin counteracts the effects of cortisol, the stress hormone. Elevated cortisol levels can lead to anxiety, depression and other health issues. The calming presence of a pet not only reduces cortisol levels but also promotes feelings of safety and comfort, creating a natural buffer against stress. A study published in the *Journal of Psychosomatic Research* found that pet owners exhibited lower levels of stress and improved overall well-being compared to non-pet owners (Allen et al., 2002).

The Therapeutic Power of Petting

The simple act of petting an animal triggers a cascade of physiological responses that promote relaxation. This repetitive motion not only provides sensory pleasure but also activates the PNS, lowering heart rate and blood pressure. Research published in the *Psychological Reports* indicates that interacting with animals can lead to a significant decrease in physiological markers of stress, such as heart rate and blood pressure (Barker et al., 2016). These changes reflect a state of relaxation and calm, essential for overall mental health.

Practical Ways to Engage with Pets for Stress Relief

- **Petting and Cuddling:** Make it a daily ritual to spend a few minutes petting your dog or cat. This simple action can significantly lower your heart rate and blood pressure. Aim for at least 15–30 minutes a day.
- **Mindful Interactions:** Focus on the texture of your pet's fur, the warmth of their body and the sounds they make. This mindfulness practice can help centre your thoughts and reduce anxiety.
- **Interactive Play:** Engage in interactive play with your pet, such as throwing a ball for your dog or using a laser pointer for your cat. Physical activity releases endorphins, which enhance mood and promote relaxation.
- **Nature Walks:** Take your pet for walks in nature. The combination of physical activity, fresh air and the presence of your pet can amplify stress-relieving benefits.

- **Create a Relaxation Space:** Designate a comfortable spot at home where you can unwind with your pet. This could include a cosy blanket and some toys. Having a specific place for relaxation can help reinforce the connection between your pet and stress relief.

Pet Therapy: An Alternative for All

For individuals unable to keep pets due to allergies, lifestyle constraints or other reasons, pet therapy offers a viable alternative. Animal-assisted therapy (AAT) involves structured interactions between individuals and trained therapy animals, often conducted in therapeutic settings. These sessions are designed to achieve specific therapeutic goals, including reducing anxiety, enhancing emotional regulation and promoting social engagement.

Therapy animals, often dogs, are specially trained to provide comfort and support to individuals in various therapeutic contexts. A study published in *Psychological Reports* highlighted that patients undergoing AAT experienced significant reductions in anxiety and depression symptoms, emphasizing the therapy animals' role in creating a supportive and calming environment (Glenk et al., 2017). The presence of a friendly, calm animal can make social interactions feel less intimidating, serving as a bridge to greater social engagement.

Practical Steps to Engage in Pet Therapy

- **Seek Professional Therapy:** Look for certified animal-assisted therapy programmes in your area. Many hospitals, schools and rehabilitation centres offer AAT sessions.
- **Volunteer with Therapy Animals:** If you are unable to have a pet at home, consider volunteering with organizations that provide therapy animals to facilities like nursing homes or hospitals. This can give you the chance to experience the calming effects of animals.

- **Participate in Group Sessions:** Join workshops or group therapy sessions that involve interaction with therapy animals. These environments can provide a structured way to engage with pets, while benefiting from group support.

The Effects of Animals on Pain Management

The effectiveness of pet therapy extends beyond emotional support; studies indicate that animals can also reduce perceptions of pain. Research published in the *Journal of Pain Medicine* found that patients exposed to therapy animals reported lower pain levels and improved emotional well-being, showcasing the distraction and relaxation that animal interactions can provide (Morrison et al., 2018).

Dr Julie Hanks, a clinical social worker and author, states, 'The unconditional love from pets provides emotional support that is healing and grounding. It builds connection in a world that often feels disconnected.'

Similarly, Dr Elizabeth Lange, a veterinarian and animal behaviourist, notes, 'The way animals engage with us can create a safe space for emotional expression. They help us feel understood, which can be a powerful tool in managing stress and anxiety.'

These insights echo the scientific findings that highlight the transformative power of pets in our lives. The loving connection we establish with animals can serve as a vital component of mental health, offering support, comfort and a sense of belonging.

So it's clear—our furry friends are not just companions; they are essential partners in our journey towards emotional health and balance.

11

Engage Your Senses Consciously

You, I and everyone in this world are connected to each other and everything in our environment through our five senses. What are they? The ability to hear, see, taste, smell and touch. These five senses are not just ways to perceive the world, rather they are our shield—defence mechanisms that protect and guide us. By actively engaging in our senses, we create a powerful pathway to return to the present moment.

The five senses do more than connecting us to our surroundings; they also provide a gateway to regulate our nervous system. In times of stress, they help us ground ourselves and shift from a state of restlessness or anxiety to one of calmness and awareness. In moments of lethargy or low mood, activating our senses can up-regulate our system, bringing us back to alertness and engagement. This concept aligns closely with studies that have examined how some of the world's happiest people stay present. In various global studies, including research on resilience and happiness, a key factor linked to well-being was the ability to stay present and connected to one's environment, especially through the senses.

As Lao Tzu's wisdom goes, 'If you are anxious, you are in the future because it is unknown. If you are full of guilt and sadness, you are in the past because nothing can change that. If you are in the now, you are happy because life is happening now.' Anchoring ourselves in the present, through our senses, is one of the most effective, science-backed methods to re-establish calmness and clarity.

Our five senses directly interact with our nervous system, constantly sending signals to the brain that help us interpret our environment. This information is processed primarily in two areas of the brain: the thalamus, which directs sensory information to appropriate regions, and the limbic system, where emotions and memories are processed. When our senses detect something alarming, the amygdala in the limbic system activates our fight-or-flight response. However, when we consciously direct our senses to non-threatening stimuli, we signal the brain that it is safe, encouraging a shift from sympathetic (fight-or-flight) to parasympathetic (rest-and-digest) mode.

Studies published by the NCBI and on PubMed have demonstrated the efficacy of sensory engagement practices in reducing stress. One study found that sensory-based mindfulness practices reduced cortisol levels and heart rate variability, indicators of reduced stress response in participants. Additionally, clinical psychologists and therapists, such as Dr Rick Hanson, author of *Hardwiring Happiness,* emphasize the importance of sensory engagement in emotional regulation, explaining that it allows us to interrupt negative thought loops and reconnect with a calming present.

Using Your Senses to Ground and Calm

Imagine you're at work, and your mind begins spiralling into a flood of anxious thoughts, pulling you into past resentments or future fears. This is where engaging in the senses, one by one, becomes a potent tool to halt the flow of negative thinking and bring you back to a stable, present moment. Let's walk through each sense, practising it with intention.

- **Sight**
  Focus on a single object in your immediate surroundings, perhaps, a pen, a cup or a plant. Study

it as if you're seeing it for the first time—notice its texture, colours and contours. This simple act of focusing on a tangible object draws your attention away from stressful thoughts and into the now.

- **Hearing**
  Tune in to one specific sound in your environment. Perhaps, it's the hum of an air conditioner, distant voices or even your own breath. The brain is wired to prioritize auditory stimuli, so, engaging this sense, with focus, can interrupt internal chatter and promote a peaceful state.
- **Smell**
  Notice any scent around you. It might be the faint whiff of coffee, a colleague's perfume or even the subtle smell of the room. Research shows that the olfactory bulb is directly connected to the amygdala, meaning that scent can significantly influence mood and memory. Scent-based mindfulness can evoke calm and pleasant memories, instantly down-regulating stress responses.
- **Taste**
  Take a moment to notice the taste in your mouth, whether it's residual from a recent meal or simply neutral. Taste is an underutilized sense in mindfulness but can be incredibly grounding. When you consciously taste something, you redirect your focus, slowing the mental chatter.
- **Touch**
  Focus on the texture of something nearby—a soft fabric, the smooth surface of a table or even your own skin. Touch is closely connected to the release of oxytocin, the 'love hormone', which reduces cortisol and boosts a sense of safety. Actively engaging in this sense signals the brain to relax, helping to down-regulate a stressed nervous system.

Engaging each sense, one at a time, is like hitting the 'reset' button on a racing mind. This approach is also referred to as the 'focused distraction method', capitalizing on the brain's poor ability to multitask. By intentionally shifting from one sense to another, we give ourselves the chance to pause, recalibrate and return to the present.

The Role of Senses in Up-regulating a Down-regulated Nervous System

While the senses play a crucial role in calming the nervous system, they can also be used to stimulate a lethargic or unmotivated state. For instance, listening to uplifting music, viewing bright colours or engaging with vibrant scents can re-energize a tired mind. Therapists often use sensory strategies for clients experiencing depression or lethargy, encouraging sensory-based routines to reawaken motivation and excitement.

Dr Dan Siegel, a clinical professor of psychiatry, speaks to the 'window of tolerance' concept, where our nervous system operates optimally. He explains that sensory engagement can be the key to expanding this window, helping us move away from either hypo-arousal (under-stimulation) or hyper-arousal (over-stimulation), towards a balanced state of alertness.

Therapists and psychologists increasingly advocate for sensory-based grounding techniques as a means of managing stress and anxiety. According to Dr Tara Brach, an expert in mindfulness psychology, sensory awareness is among the most effective tools for grounding because it requires minimal effort and can be used anywhere. Brach explains that by concentrating on the sensory experience, we remove the emotional charge from stressful situations, allowing the brain to process the experience in a safer context.

A growing body of research, including studies published on platforms like PubMed, supports the use of sensory engagement for trauma-informed therapy and stress regulation. Patients in these studies have reported reduced symptoms of anxiety, decreased heart rate and increased feelings of safety and connection when engaging in sensory exercises.

Sensory engagement does more than calm us down in times of stress. When practised regularly, it builds resilience, helping us handle future stressors with greater ease. Many therapists liken this practice to a 'mental gym', where each sensory exercise strengthens our ability to stay present, manage emotions and improve our relationship with stress.

Our five senses serve as powerful allies for anchoring us to the present, regulating the nervous system and enhancing our overall well-being. In times of stress, activating each sense mindfully can help down-regulate our nervous system, bringing calmness and clarity. When energy or motivation is lacking, sensory stimulation can lift us back to a state of engagement. Engaging the senses is a timeless and scientifically supported practice for finding balance, resilience and a greater sense of presence in our day-to-day lives.

12

Make Light of a Situation

What if I told you that one of the most effective strategies for regulating our nervous system and keeping stress at bay is simply learning to make light of a situation and not sweat the small stuff?

I often reflect on my encounters with centenarians—remarkable individuals who embody the beauty of a life well-lived. These wise souls, ranging from their seventies to their hundreds, have a unique perspective on life that often revolves around humour. One particularly unforgettable moment was with a ninety-six-year-old man at a gathering. He was standing tall and laughing heartily, a beacon of joy and vitality. When I asked him about the secret to his longevity, he simply said, 'I don't take things too seriously.' This profound wisdom struck me deeply.

He acknowledged that, like everyone, he faced challenges. However, his approach was refreshing: feel the emotions, but don't dwell on them. If a situation allows it, 'shake things up by just loosening up and making light of it'. This perspective is a profound reminder that life doesn't have to be a serious affair.

The Art of Letting Go

How often do we find ourselves overwhelmed by challenges that seem insurmountable? We wear our emotions like heavy coats, letting the slightest setback rattle us. Psychologist

Dr Robert Sapolsky, in his insightful book *Why Zebras Don't Get Ulcers*, explains that prolonged stress can lead to various health issues, including anxiety and heart disease. Yet, by adopting a relaxed perspective and learning to let go, we can transform our experience of stress.

When we make light of situations, we shift our perspective. Instead of viewing challenges as threats, we begin to see them as opportunities for growth or, at the very least, sources of keeping things light-hearted. Dr Norman Cousins, author of *Anatomy of an Illness*, demonstrated the healing power of humour through his personal journey with a serious illness. He documented how watching comedies and laughing helped him alleviate severe pain and improve his overall health. His experience illustrates that laughter is not just a response; it can be a powerful remedy.

A Lesson from the Wise

One of the most significant lessons from the centenarians I meet is the art of letting go. They possess an incredible ability to face adversity with grace and humour, embracing the unpredictability of life. Psychologist Dr Brené Brown, in her book *Daring Greatly*, emphasizes the importance of vulnerability and letting go of perfectionism. She posits that embracing imperfection allows us to live wholeheartedly, creating a sense of connection and belonging.

By letting go of our attachment to outcomes and choosing to respond with humour, we create a pathway to peace. This shift not only benefits our mental health but also contributes to our physical well-being. Dr Herbert Benson, in *The Relaxation Response*, highlights how relaxation techniques—including humour—induce physiological changes that promote healing and reduce stress.

Ready to infuse your life with laughter and light-heartedness? Here are some practical strategies:

1. **Find Humour in Everyday Situations:** Cultivate the habit of looking for the funny side of daily challenges.

Whether it's a minor mishap or an unexpected setback, allow yourself to laugh at the absurdity of life.

2. **Surround Yourself with Positive People:** Spend time with those who uplift you and inspire laughter. Their positive energy can help you cultivate a lighter perspective on life.
3. **Practise Mindfulness:** Mindfulness helps you become aware of your thoughts and feelings without judgement. Recognizing when you're taking things too seriously allows you to consciously choose a lighter response.
4. **Engage in Playful Activities:** Embrace activities that bring you joy and laughter, whether it's playing games, watching comedies or participating in creative pursuits. Allow yourself the freedom to play.
5. **Reflect on Your Perspective:** Regularly check in with yourself about what truly matters. Are you holding onto stress over trivial matters? Challenge yourself to let go and focus on what brings you joy.

Making light of a situation and not sweating the small stuff are essential practices for maintaining a balanced nervous system and reducing stress levels. By letting go of seriousness, and shifting our perspective, we cultivate resilience and create space for joy in our lives. The wisdom of centenarians reminds us that life is too short to take everything to heart.

So, let's choose to laugh, let go and enjoy the journey. After all, the secret to a vibrant, healthy life may very well lie in our ability to find humour amidst the chaos. As you navigate through life's challenges, remember: sometimes, all you need is a little laughter to lighten the load.

13

Giving Back and Service

Giving back is not only a beautiful act of kindness but also a profound tool for calming and balancing our nervous system. Serving others enables us to shift from an overactive sympathetic state (fight-or-flight) to the soothing parasympathetic state (rest-and-digest). Research has shown that engaging in acts of service can help regulate stress responses, creating a deep sense of peace and satisfaction that contributes to mental, emotional and physical well-being.

Science of Service

Scientific studies highlight the healing power of service, demonstrating how it benefits both the giver and the receiver. According to research, selfless acts stimulate areas of the brain associated with pleasure and reward, such as the mesolimbic system, releasing dopamine, oxytocin and endorphins. These neurochemicals help reduce stress, combat anxiety and enhance mood, creating a 'helper's high'. The experience is so powerful that it has been shown to reduce symptoms of depression and even enhance longevity.

Experts in psychology and neuroscience underscore that the positive emotions we feel, when giving, are transformative. Dr Stephen Porges, a prominent neuroscientist and creator of the Polyvagal Theory, explains that engaging in socially connected acts, like helping others, enhances vagal tone, a measure of the health of our PNS.

Improved vagal tone is linked to reduced inflammation, better heart health and an overall calming of the body's stress response, enabling us to shift into a balanced, restorative state.

Giving from the Heart: True Service Without Expectation

The fulfilment derived from giving reaches its peak when we act without expectation. This idea resonates deeply with the concept of non-transactional relationships—serving because we want to, not because we want something in return. Service from the heart is the kind that can't be bought with money. It's about offering a part of ourselves, whether it's our time, attention, knowledge or simply a listening ear. Everyone can serve, no matter who they are or what they do. You don't need a medical degree or a special title; what matters most is the sincerity behind your actions.

Service also enables us to connect with a sense of greatness that far surpasses fleeting fame or recognition. While fame can feel empty, true greatness is rooted in helping others, and it brings a satisfaction that sustains us over time. Service helps cultivate humility, gratitude and empathy, grounding us in a greater purpose. By serving those around us—whether family, friends, strangers or even the planet—we nurture these qualities within ourselves, bringing balance and fulfilment.

Simple Acts with Profound Effects

The beauty of service lies in its simplicity. Small acts of kindness can have significant impacts on both our nervous system and our well-being. Volunteer your time, mentor someone or lend a compassionate ear. Even offering kindness to strangers can transform your day, reinforcing a positive cycle of giving and receiving.

Personally, I have felt this deep joy during my time donating plasma for children with cancer at the Tata Memorial

Hospital. For the past two years, I've given my time, travelled and donated my blood to support these young lives. In return, I feel an immense sense of fulfilment, knowing that I have played a small role. Every donation is a reminder that while giving takes energy, it also restores, revitalizing us in a way that nothing else can.

Similarly, in my work, I strive to serve my patients daily, alongside my team. Yes, we receive compensation, like any job, but what truly fuels us is seeing the lives we touch and transform. When a patient approaches us or writes to say, 'You changed my life,' it fills our hearts beyond measure. The sense of purpose and joy we gain from these heartfelt moments is something no monetary reward could ever replace.

Giving also cultivates a continuous flow of positive energy. Just as love and knowledge are meant to be shared, so is our compassion. In relationships, we often begin by giving love freely but later place conditions on it. When we learn to love without strings attached, we maintain a steady flow of positive energy that strengthens our connections and benefits our own well-being.

This principle applies to money and material wealth as well. While it's natural to want financial security, hoarding wealth can create stagnation. Many affluent individuals experience profound joy when they share their resources, not just in grand gestures but also through simple acts of generosity. It's a reminder that true abundance comes from sharing our blessings with others.

Numerous studies confirm the mental and physical health benefits of giving. A report from the Greater Good Science Center at UC Berkeley notes that giving increases life satisfaction, enhances social bonds and even boosts immune function. When we contribute to others' well-being, our bodies release oxytocin, which promotes bonding, trust and feelings of safety. This effect is especially powerful for individuals who experience high levels of stress, as giving has been shown to buffer against stress-related health problems.

In a study published in *Psychosomatic Medicine,* researchers found that participants who provided social support to others had lower mortality rates than those who didn't. This study highlights the powerful link between giving and longevity. Engaging in altruistic acts appears to reduce the negative effects of stress, especially in high-stress environments, and improve overall health outcomes.

Ways to Start Giving Back

You don't need to be a professional or a certified expert to give back. Anyone can contribute in their own unique way, offering their time, presence and compassion. Here are a few ideas to get started:

- **Offer Time and Space:** Listen to someone in need, offer support and give your time genuinely.
- **Share Skills and Knowledge:** Teach or mentor someone in a skill you excel at, whether it's cooking, painting or yoga.
- **Practise Kindness and Compassion:** Simple acts of kindness, such as helping a neighbour or offering words of encouragement, make a difference.
- **Serve the Planet:** Consider eco-friendly initiatives, like planting trees, reducing waste or supporting sustainable practices.
- **Volunteer for a Cause:** Find a cause that resonates with you and dedicate a few hours each month to making a difference.

In the end, the energy of giving flows both ways. When you give freely and with an open heart, it nourishes your soul and uplifts others. In its purest form, giving back is a powerful tool for personal healing and fulfilment. When done selflessly, it taps into the deepest, most meaningful aspects of our humanity, offering us a way to make a lasting difference in the world while nurturing our own hearts. Start today and experience the joy and peace that only giving back can bring.

14

Grounding Exercises/Barefoot Connections/Walks

In today's technology-driven world, it's all too easy to feel disconnected—not just from nature, but from ourselves. We live in concrete structures, step on asphalt and wear shoes that often shield us from direct contact with the Earth. Yet, there is a simple, powerful practice that can restore this lost connection and help us find a sense of calm: grounding, or earthing.

Grounding exercises involve making direct physical contact with the Earth's surface, like walking barefoot on grass, soil or sand, and can play a crucial role in moving our nervous system from a state of 'fight-or-flight' to 'rest-and-digest'.

Grounding is not a new concept. For centuries, our ancestors walked barefoot or wore rudimentary footwear that kept them connected to the Earth's energy. Simple wooden sandals, or *khadau*, were common in India, while many indigenous cultures worldwide moved barefoot across diverse terrains. This contact with the Earth was not only practical but also therapeutic—a natural way to soothe and balance the body's energy. Today, our advanced footwear often insulates us from the Earth's natural energies, yet the benefits of this direct connection remain timeless.

The Science Behind Grounding

From a scientific perspective, grounding offers health benefits, particularly when it comes to regulating the nervous system. Research has shown that direct contact with the Earth allows the body to absorb electrons from the ground, which play a critical role in neutralizing free radicals and reducing inflammation in the body. These electrons act as antioxidants, protecting our cells and supporting our immune system.

Here's how grounding impacts us on a physiological level:

- **Reduces Inflammation and Pain**
  Studies published on PubMed have highlighted that grounding can reduce inflammation in the body. Free radicals are highly reactive molecules that can damage cells and lead to inflammation, pain and various chronic conditions. By absorbing electrons from the Earth, our body gains antioxidant-like benefits, which helps neutralize these free radicals, reducing inflammation and pain. This process also helps regulate blood flow, lowering blood pressure and promoting heart health.
- **Lowers Cortisol and Promotes a Calmer State**
  Chronic stress can cause elevated cortisol levels, a hormone associated with the 'fight-or-flight' response. Elevated cortisol, over long periods, can contribute to anxiety, insomnia and an overactive nervous system. Grounding has been shown to reduce cortisol levels significantly, allowing the body to shift from sympathetic (stressed) to parasympathetic (relaxed) mode. Studies on PubMed and by NCBI have found that grounding activities, such as barefoot walking, are linked to decreased cortisol production, which naturally relaxes the body and mind.
- **Stabilizes the Body's Bioelectrical Environment**
  Our bodies operate as bioelectrical systems. The heart, brain and nervous system generate electrical impulses that control bodily functions. Grounding

helps stabilize this bioelectrical environment by recharging the body with electrons. This connection to the Earth can enhance mood, improve sleep and increase resilience to stress, making it a valuable tool for nervous system regulation.

- **Improves Sleep and Circadian Rhythm**
  Research suggests that grounding can improve sleep by regulating the body's circadian rhythm. Poor sleep can disrupt the nervous system, making us more susceptible to stress and anxiety. Grounding helps align our internal biological clock with natural rhythms, leading to deeper, restorative sleep. This connection with nature's cycles helps our body restore balance, creating a sense of calm that can support overall mental well-being.

While walking barefoot everywhere may not be feasible, incorporating designated grounding activities into your routine can make a significant difference in how you feel.

- **Walk on Clean Grass**
  Find a safe, clean patch of grass in your garden or a nearby park. Spend 15–30 minutes walking or standing barefoot, allowing your skin to absorb the Earth's electrons. You might notice a subtle sense of calm washing over you as your body syncs with the Earth's natural rhythm.
- **Walk Barefoot on the Beach**
  Beaches offer an ideal grounding experience due to the conductive properties of wet sand. As you walk along the shore, the unique texture of the sand and the natural negative ions in the environment work together to support your nervous system, helping you move into a calm, parasympathetic state.
- **Use Grounding Mats**
  If outdoor grounding isn't feasible, grounding mats can be a helpful alternative. These devices simulate the effects of walking barefoot by connecting you to the

Earth's energy indoors. Grounding mats have become popular in urban areas, providing a practical way to benefit from grounding even in indoor settings.

- **Engage in Grounding Yoga**
  Certain yoga poses, like *Tadasana* (Mountain Pose) and *Vrikshasana* (Tree Pose), are known for their grounding effects. By standing firmly on the ground and focusing on balance, these poses help cultivate a deep connection with the Earth, promoting stability and a sense of rootedness.

I visit Soneva Fushi, a barefoot luxury resort in the Maldives, often, and it's one of my favourite getaways. Every time I go there, I get to experience the effect of being largely shoe-free. From the moment you enter, you are encouraged to deposit your shoes and enjoy a week of walking barefoot on soft sand. The natural, unrestricted movement feel therapeutic. By the end of the week, the mere thought of wearing shoes seem unnecessary, almost unnatural. This experience is a reminder for me that our connection to the Earth is as natural as breathing, and often requires nothing more than removing our shoes.

Several studies reinforce the health benefits of grounding:

- **Earthing (Grounding) Improves Sleep and Reduces Pain and Stress**
  A pivotal study published on PubMed found that grounding could improve sleep quality, reduce pain and lower stress levels in participants. This aligns with the idea that grounding can lower cortisol and support a shift to the parasympathetic nervous state, reducing anxiety and promoting overall wellness.
- **Electrons from the Earth as Natural Antioxidants**
  Research on grounding, published by NCBI, revealed that the Earth's electrons play a vital role in neutralizing

oxidative stress in the body. This scientific basis for grounding explains why it's effective for inflammation reduction, pain relief and the promotion of calmness.

- **Grounding and Blood Flow**
  Another study found that grounding improves circulation by positively influencing the red blood cells and reducing blood viscosity, which is linked to cardiovascular health. This effect has shown promise for individuals with chronic stress and high blood pressure, as it enhances blood flow and relaxation.

Whether it's a barefoot walk on the beach, grounding yoga or simply standing on grass, grounding can be woven into our lives as a powerful act of self-care. So, the next time you feel overwhelmed or unbalanced, remember that calmness might be as simple as stepping outside, kicking off your shoes and reconnecting with the Earth beneath you.

15

A Warm Cup of Tea, Soup or Coffee

There's something universally comforting about a warm cup of tea, soup or coffee. Isn't it? Maybe it's the soothing warmth radiating through your hands, or the gentle steam filling the air with aromas that feel like a cosy hug. When you're feeling under the weather—physically or emotionally—a warm drink or a hot bowl of soup can do more than just warm you up; it can lift your spirits and bring back memories of simpler times, reconnecting us to something timeless and deeply personal.

The Science of Warmth: How Temperature Affects Us

Studies have shown that warm drinks affect the body and mind. A study from Yale University, for instance, discovered that holding a warm beverage could increase feelings of interpersonal warmth—essentially making us feel more positive and connected to others (Williams and Bargh, 2008). Psychologically, warmth is linked with comfort and empathy.

On a physical level, warm drinks and foods help the body conserve energy. When we drink or eat warm substances, our body doesn't have to expend as much energy to heat them, which can be especially comforting during cold weather or when you're unwell. This effect is well-documented in research on thermoregulation, where internal warmth helps stimulate the PNS, putting the body in a rest-and-digest state that counters stress and anxiety.

Warm Tea: Comfort in a Cup

In India, tea is synonymous with childhood memories for many. Imagine grandmothers brewing fragrant, spiced chai every afternoon, pouring it into tiny clay cups and sitting in the courtyard as the sun dipped behind the trees. Tea has a long history as a remedy, not just for the body but also for the spirit. Whether it's ginger tea for nausea, peppermint for digestion or chamomile to calm the nerves, every culture seems to have its version of tea therapy. In Ayurveda and traditional Chinese medicine, warm tea is believed to balance the body's energy and support digestion, thus calming the mind while nurturing the body.

Scientific studies back these traditional beliefs. A study published in *Psychopharmacology*, in 2012, found that the amino acid L-theanine, naturally present in green tea, has anti-stress effects, reducing cortisol levels and promoting relaxation without drowsiness (Wakabayashi et al., 2012). The antioxidants in tea can also help reduce inflammation and improve immune function, making it a go-to drink.

Warm Soup: Nourishment and Nostalgia

Soup is another remedy rooted in tradition. Imagine a warm bowl of soup, fragrant with spices and bursting with fresh herbs, when you feel sick.

Beyond nostalgia, soup has physiological benefits. Broth-based soups can help replenish electrolytes and hydrate the body, which are vital when you feel drained. Chicken soup, commonly known as a remedy for colds, has been studied for its mild anti-inflammatory effects. A study from the University of Nebraska Medical Center found that chicken soup inhibits the movement of neutrophils—white blood cells that are part of the immune system response to infection—reducing cold symptoms and aiding in faster recovery (Rennard et al., 2000).

Warm soup also has a vasodilatory effect, which means it helps open up blood vessels, allowing better circulation and warmth distribution throughout the body. This effect can help alleviate aches and pains, enhancing its healing power.

Warm Coffee: Energizing the Spirit

I remember my first sip of coffee—a simple, dark brew. It was bitter but there was something about the ritual of it, the break and the warmth it offered. Over the years, I have had several amazing conversations over mugs of coffee. When I first decided to quit corporate life and answer my calling of practising integrative and lifestyle medicine, for a long time, I operated out of cafes. The memories associated with it, make it special. I love my coffee and exploring cafes on my trips. Coffee, with its stimulating effects, is not just a drink but also, often, a reason to pause, reflect and connect, provided you have the right quality and quantity.

Studies published in the *Journal of Alzheimer's Disease* show that moderate coffee consumption is linked with improved mood and mental alertness (Lara, 2010). Caffeine blocks adenosine, a neurotransmitter that makes us feel tired, thus promoting wakefulness. However, the ritual of holding a warm mug and inhaling the earthy aroma also releases dopamine, creating a sense of pleasure and satisfaction.

Coffee's effect isn't just chemical; it's cultural. Coffee houses have historically been gathering places, where people come to connect and converse. These places serve not just coffee but also a sense of community, which can be deeply healing in times of isolation.

When you sip on warm tea, soup or coffee, you naturally slow down and savour the moment. This mindfulness practice can lower your stress and anxiety levels, thereby promoting relaxation.

Make this ritual more effective by:

- Creating a relaxing environment. Enjoy your warm beverage or soup in a quiet, comfortable setting.
- Focus on the experience—savour the flavours, warmth and aroma.

- The next time you're feeling stressed, try brewing a cup of herbal tea or warming up some soup. Take a moment to breathe deeply, feel the warmth and let your body relax. Invite a friend over for coffee, or enjoy your tea in a cosy corner with a good book. These small, mindful practices can make a big difference in how you feel.

In moments when we feel disconnected or lonely, a warm cup or bowl can help bridge that gap, reminding us of the warmth we carry from past generations. Whether you prefer tea, coffee or soup, remember that the warmth isn't just in the drink or the food—it's in the memories, the love and the comfort they carry with them.

16

The Power of a Hug

Have you ever noticed that when a child is being naughty and is scolded by their mother, their first instinct—despite being upset—is to run back into her arms for a hug? It's an almost magical reaction, one that shows just how deeply wired our need for safety and comfort is. The child may be upset, even crying, but instinctively turns to the very person who just corrected them.

Hugs provide emotional regulation. For a child, a mother's embrace offers warmth, security and reassurance even when they are upset. The physical act of hugging activates the PNS, which helps calm the body's stress response. In that moment, the hug becomes a healing balm, offering relief from confusion or hurt feelings. Even if they don't fully understand the situation, a child feels protected, loved and accepted through the simple act of touch.

Psychologically, this moment of connection helps the child make sense of their emotions. It's as though they're saying, 'I may have been wrong, but I know I'm safe with you.' Studies in *Infant Behavior and Development* show that when children seek physical contact, it's their way of self-soothing—they turn to their caregiver because they innately understand that closeness will help them feel better (Bigelow and Williams, 2020).

A mother's hug or any caregiver's embrace acts as an emotional anchor for the child. It helps them navigate their big, confusing emotions, while reinforcing the deep bond of trust that they rely on. In a world that can sometimes feel overwhelming or scary, a hug represents stability and unconditional love, offering them the safety to express their feelings and eventually move past them. The next time you notice a child seeking comfort through a hug, remember that it's more than just a physical act.

This need for touch is not exclusive to children, though it is most evident in them. As adults, we, too, crave that sense of safety and connection through touch. The hug that soothes a child can do the same for us, helping us feel grounded and supported in moments of stress or emotional overwhelm. Let's dive into this, shall we?

Stressed? Feeling down? Drained? Sometimes, the solution isn't a cup of coffee or a walk outside—it's as simple as a hug. A deep, consensual hug from a loved one can work wonders for your body and mind, shifting you from stress to serenity in just 20 seconds.

The Twenty-Second Hug: A Simple Act with Big Benefits

Research published in *Behavioral Medicine* shows that a twenty-second hug has profound physiological effects, particularly by activating the PNS—the part of your body that helps you relax and recover from stress (Grewen et al., 2003).

How to Enjoy a Twenty-Second Hug:

1. **Choose someone special:** This could be a family member, friend or loved one.
2. **Find comfort:** Whether standing or sitting, embrace fully so that both of you feel comfortable and secure.
3. **Hold the hug:** Maintain the embrace for at least 20 seconds. This might feel longer than usual, but the results are worth it.

4. **Breathe together:** Focus on deep breathing, inhaling through your nose and exhaling slowly through your mouth. Synchronize your breaths for an even deeper connection.

Why It Works: The Science Behind Hugging

The act of embracing has immense effects. Here's what happens to your body during and after a good hug.

When you hug someone for more than a few seconds, your body releases oxytocin, commonly known as the love or cuddle hormone. This amazing chemical has a cascade of benefits:

- **Reduces cortisol levels:** Cortisol, the stress hormone, decreases significantly, helping to relieve stress and anxiety.
- **Lowers heart rate and blood pressure:** Studies have shown that hugging can have immediate calming effects on the cardiovascular system.
- **Boosts feelings of trust and security:** Oxytocin creates a sense of emotional closeness and connection.
- **Releases endorphins:** These natural painkillers create a sense of well-being and even help alleviate physical discomfort.

A study published in *Psychological Science* found that people who received more hugs were less likely to get sick after being exposed to a virus. This suggests that hugs could actually bolster your immune system! (Cohen et al., 2015.)

Self-Hugging: The Ultimate Act of Self-Compassion

However, what if you're alone? Enter the self-hug. While it may sound unconventional, self-hugging has been shown to offer many of the same benefits as embracing another person. It's a powerful way to cultivate self-love, reduce stress and remind yourself that you're worthy of care—even from yourself.

How to Do a Self-Hug:

1. **Sit or stand comfortably:** Place your arms across your body, with each hand resting on the opposite shoulder or bicep.
2. **Apply gentle pressure:** Squeeze your arms around yourself and hold the position for 20 seconds. Focus on the warmth and safety of your own touch.
3. **Breathe deeply:** As with a traditional hug, concentrate on slow, steady breathing.

Self-hugging activates interoception, your body's awareness of its internal state. This practice can calm the nervous system and bring a sense of emotional regulation. A study published in *Frontiers in Psychology* found that self-hugging could reduce your perception of pain, similar to how physical touch from others provides relief (Uvnäs-Moberg, Handlin, and Petersson, 2015).

The Power of Touch: Why We Crave Connection

Human beings are wired for connection. Touch, particularly hugging, plays a big role in our emotional and physical well-being. In fact, researchers at the Touch Research Institute at the University of Miami found that even gentle forms of touch—like holding hands or a pat on the back—can reduce symptoms of depression, lower stress and even improve sleep (Field, 2010).

Hugging is one of the most intimate forms of touch, which is why its benefits run so deep. In a world where we often rely on screens for communication, the simple act of holding someone close can bring us back to the essentials of human connection.

Hugging Tips: Make the Most of Every Embrace

1. **Take your time:** Don't rush. The magic of hugging lies in its ability to calm and ground you, and a few extra seconds can make all the difference.
2. **Be fully present:** Put away distractions, like your phone, and focus on the warmth of the embrace.
3. **Synchronize your breath:** For a deeper emotional connection, try breathing in sync with the person you're hugging.
4. **Initiate a hug when needed:** Hugs don't always have to be reactive. If someone seems stressed, a simple embrace can be exactly what they need.

So, what are you waiting for? Whether you're with a loved one or practising a self-hug, take 20 seconds right now and give yourself the gift of calmness, connection and care. Hugging is the simplest, yet most profound, way to de-stress, connect and heal. Try it today. Do it well.

17

Memories and Recalling Happy Moments

Imagine scrolling through your Facebook or Instagram feed when, suddenly, a familiar image from a cherished moment in your past appears before you. It might be a picture of a sun-soaked beach day with friends, a birthday celebration or a quiet moment with a loved one. Instantly, your heart warms, and a smile crosses your face as a flood of nostalgia washes over you. This is the beauty of memories—a unique portal that transports us back to moments that light up our hearts and lift our spirits.

The Neuroscience of Memory

To understand the healing potential of memories, we must explore the neuroscience behind them. When we recall positive and uplifting experiences, specific areas of our brains are activated. The **hippocampus** is crucial for forming and retrieving memories, while the **amygdala** processes the emotions associated with these memories.

According to research published in *Psychological Science*, the amygdala not only helps to encode emotional memories but also influences how we recall them later, highlighting the intimate connection between emotion and memory (LaBar and Phelps, 1998).

When we think about happy memories, our brains release **neurotransmitters** such as **dopamine** and **serotonin**. These chemicals play vital roles in regulating mood, emotions and overall well-being. A study in *Psychopharmocology* indicates that engaging in activities, which evoke positive memories, can increase dopamine levels, significantly contributing to feelings of pleasure and reward (Berridge and Kringelbach, 2008).

Changes in the Brain and Body

The process of recalling happy memories triggers a cascade of physiological responses in our bodies:

1. **Amygdala Activation:** When we think of a positive memory, the amygdala becomes active, modulating emotional responses. This area is key to how we experience joy, love and happiness, and its engagement can mitigate the negative effects of stress. Research published in *Current Opinion in Neurobiology* emphasizes that the emotional significance of memories is crucial for how we perceive and respond to our experiences (Phelps et al., 2004).
2. **Neurotransmitter Release:** Recalling uplifting memories leads to the release of neurotransmitters like dopamine, serotonin and oxytocin. Dopamine is associated with feelings of pleasure and reward, while serotonin helps stabilize mood. Oxytocin, often dubbed the 'bonding hormone', enhances feelings of connection and trust, making us feel more secure. A study in *Social Cognitive and Affective Neuroscience* highlights oxytocin's role in building social connections and emotional well-being (Hein and Silani, 2008).
3. **Reduction in Cortisol Levels:** Positive memory recall can lower cortisol levels in the body. Cortisol, known as the stress hormone, is elevated during periods of anxiety and stress. Lowering cortisol not only reduces feelings of stress but also promotes overall health by decreasing the risk of stress-related illnesses. Research in *Psychoneuroendocrinology* shows that engaging

with positive memories can help regulate cortisol, leading to improved mental health outcomes (Mills et al., 2015).

4. **Enhanced Immune Function**: Research has shown that positive emotions can boost immune function, helping the body to resist illnesses better. A study published in *Psychosomatic Medicine* found that individuals, who frequently engaged in positive reminiscing, exhibited stronger immune responses, highlighting the link between emotional well-being and physical health (Cohen et al., 2003).
5. **Physical Relaxation**: Recalling happy memories can lead to a decrease in muscle tension and an overall sense of relaxation. This physical response is crucial for transitioning from a state of stress to one of calm and safety.

In Integrative and Lifestyle Medicine, our focus extends beyond nutrition, exercise and sleep; we also emphasize the importance of simple lifestyle changes that can significantly enrich our patients' lives. One powerful technique that we employ is the 'memory gallery' approach. This method encourages individuals to visualize a gallery filled with snapshots of their happiest moments. When they encounter stress or anxiety, we invite our patients to 'visit' this gallery, pausing at a specific 'happy picture'. Here, they immerse themselves in the vivid details of that memory—the sights, sounds, smells and emotions associated with those joyful moments. This practice not only evokes positive feelings but also serves as a powerful remedy for shifting from distress to a state of calm and safety.

We also work with patients in palliative care, who often return home after all medical options have been exhausted. Among the various strategies that we employ to enhance their quality of life and alleviate suffering, we encourage these individuals to reflect on their cherished memories. This practice, known as reminiscence therapy, proves to be profoundly impactful. It is heart-warming to witness how recalling moments filled with love, joy and connection can illuminate their eyes and hearts, providing solace amid suffering. Such reflections often become a source of strength, allowing patients to find joy in the present, even in the face of adversity. Engaging with photo albums or sharing stories from the past transforms these experiences into a powerful medicine for the soul.

Creating lasting memories with our children and loved ones is crucial for all of us. There is much to learn from our end-of-life patients. In conversations with them, they seldom mention accolades, brands or social media followers they earned through their lifetime. Instead, they treasure the memories they have created and shared with loved ones. They reminisce about shared laughter, family gatherings and heartfelt conversations—beautiful memories that provide comfort and a sense of safety during challenging times.

Memories are not merely fragments of our past; they are medicinal for our emotional health and state of mind.

18

Raising Our Vibrations

Everything in the universe, from a tiny atom to the largest galaxy, vibrates at a unique frequency, and human beings are no different. In scientific terms, 'vibration' refers to the frequency at which our cells, thoughts and emotions oscillate. Each cell in our body has a distinct frequency, and collectively, these frequencies create an overall vibrational state that influences our health and well-being. In our daily experiences, this vibration influences how we feel physically, emotionally and mentally. Higher vibrations—such as feelings of love, joy and compassion—are energizing and life-enhancing, while lower vibrations—like sadness, anger or stress—often make us feel drained and unwell.

The field of psychoneuroimmunology, which studies the connection between thoughts, the nervous system and immunity, has shown that high vibrational states can promote healing, increase resilience and improve immune function. When our thoughts and actions align with higher vibrational frequencies, our body releases feel-good neurotransmitters, like dopamine and serotonin, which create feelings of happiness and contentment. Conversely, staying in low-vibration states, such as chronic stress or sadness, can elevate cortisol, the body's main stress hormone, which may weaken immunity and increase inflammation.

How Raising Vibrations Affects the Nervous System

Raising our vibration helps to activate the PNS, shifting us from a state of stress and alertness to one of calmness and relaxation. Studies on PubMed and by the NCBI have shown that activities, which elevate our vibrations—such as practising gratitude, listening to uplifting music or connecting with loved ones—can help move us from the SNS to the PNS. This shift creates space for the body to rest, recover and promote healing.

Are Vibes Real? Understanding Subtle Energy and Human Perception

You might have experienced entering a room after an argument has taken place, even though everyone has already left. Somehow, you still sense an underlying tension, as if something lingers in the air. Or, perhaps, you've felt an inexplicable warmth and comfort when meeting someone who radiates positivity, even if you've only just met them. These 'vibes' are real and often reflect the energy and emotions present in our surroundings.

Scientific studies reveal that humans are sensitive to these subtle energetic shifts, which influence our mood and physiological responses. In stressful environments, cortisol levels can rise, triggering our SNS and potentially dampening our mood. In contrast, being around positive people can release oxytocin—the 'bonding hormone'—which makes us feel relaxed, happy and connected. We pick up on each other's energy unconsciously, just as we sense someone's joy or sadness without them saying a word.

The music we listen to also affects our vibrational state. If someone is going through a difficult break-up, they may find comfort in listening to sad music that resonates with their emotional state, yet, staying in that low vibration can hinder recovery. On the other hand, upbeat music can quickly raise their spirits, releasing dopamine and lifting their mood. Likewise, spending time with children or animals, who naturally vibrate at high frequencies, often brings us joy and relaxation because their presence has an inherently calming effect.

Practical Ways to Raise Your Vibrations

Raising your vibrational frequency doesn't require big, dramatic changes. Small, everyday actions can significantly influence how you feel, helping you shift from stress and anxiety to a state of peace, joy and relaxation. Here are some practical techniques:

1. **Smile at others, even if it's forced:** Smiling, even when it doesn't feel genuine, can trigger the release of dopamine, serotonin and endorphins—neurotransmitters that elevate your mood and create a ripple effect, positively influencing those around you.
2. **Laugh it out:** Laughter has a profound effect on reducing stress hormones like cortisol. It also activates the PNS, helping to calm the mind and bringing a sense of joy and ease.
3. **Pray and wish well for others:** Research shows that engaging in acts of compassion and goodwill releases oxytocin, a hormone that enhances emotional resilience and promotes feelings of warmth and connection.
4. **Be of service to others:** Helping someone else can elevate your vibration by providing a sense of purpose and fulfilment, which helps shift your focus from self-centred concerns to the well-being of others.
5. **Engage in random acts of kindness:** Simple actions like complimenting a stranger, buying a coffee for someone else or holding the door open are proven ways to boost your mood and promote a sense of interconnectedness, enhancing overall vibrational frequency.
6. **Listen to soulful music:** Music can shift brainwave patterns and activate the PNS, helping to move from

stress to calmness. Songs that resonate emotionally can have a powerful effect on raising vibrations.

7. **Spend time in nature:** Nature exposure has been linked with a reduction in cortisol levels, activating the PNS and raising vibrational frequency. Time in green spaces builds a sense of inner peace and balance, grounding and refreshing the spirit.
8. **Practise gratitude:** Studies have shown that gratitude enhances mental health, lowers stress and increases serotonin, all contributing to higher vibrational energy.
9. **Be kind and mindful with your words:** Words carry energy too. Speaking kindly and thoughtfully can uplift your own energy and create a positive atmosphere for those around you.

As you practise these simple techniques, you'll find that you feel more connected, centred and at ease. Raising your vibrations helps you develop resilience and emotional balance, allowing your mind and body to work together in harmony.

19

Cloud Gazing

Have you ever taken a moment to just lie down, look up at the sky and observe the clouds? Cloud gazing is more than a leisurely pastime; it's a scientifically supported practice that helps regulate our nervous system. Beyond the visual pleasure of drifting clouds, the act of cloud gazing invites mindfulness, meditative stillness and even a sense of emotional release.

The Science Behind Cloud Gazing

When we gaze at clouds, we activate a profound relaxation response. Cloud gazing encourages mindfulness—a meditative practice that involves bringing our full awareness to the present moment. Studies show that mindfulness can activate the PNS, reducing stress hormones like cortisol and increasing 'feel-good' neurotransmitters such as serotonin and dopamine (*JAMA*, 2014). As we lie on our backs and observe the clouds, our mind's focus shifts away from everyday stressors and distractions, bringing us into the here and now. This immersive experience in nature creates a mental shift from overthinking to simply observing, thus helping calm the mind and body.

Visual Relaxation and Reduced Mental Load

When we look at clouds, we're engaging in what scientists call 'visual relaxation'. Unlike the constant screen-based focus required by modern life, looking at clouds is a distant, passive activity that relaxes the eye muscles and reduces mental strain. Research shows that such 'soft fascination' activities—those that gently capture attention without intense focus—have a calming effect on the brain. Dr Rachel Kaplan, an environmental psychologist, describes this as 'attention restoration', which replenishes our mental energy and enhances focus.

Physical and Neurological Benefits

The act of cloud gazing engages areas of the brain linked with relaxation and pleasure, particularly the prefrontal cortex. Studies show that natural scenery, especially sky-gazing, triggers brain regions associated with positive emotions and reduces activity in the amygdala, the brain's stress centre (*Annals of the New York Academy of Sciences*). This dual relaxation of the body and mind allows us to enter a parasympathetic state, promoting deeper breathing, lowering blood pressure and, ultimately, enhancing immune function.

The Metaphor of Clouds and Emotional Release

Clouds, constantly shifting and evolving, serve as a metaphor for the transient nature of thoughts and emotions. When we see our thoughts as clouds, they become impermanent, passing experiences that we can let go of without attachment. For instance, just as a dark storm cloud eventually dissipates, so, too, can a stressful or negative thought. This practice of non-attachment is a core component of mindfulness and emotional regulation, teaching us to let go of emotions that do not serve us.

Dr Lisa Feldman Barrett, a leading psychologist, notes that when we learn to observe our emotions without judgement, we gain control over our responses. Observing clouds with a sense of detachment can have a similar effect, as we learn to witness our emotions rather than react to them. Studies published on *Perspectives on Psychological Science* affirm that practices involving non-attachment to thoughts can reduce anxiety and increase mental clarity.

Cloud gazing combines the benefits of being outdoors with the calming effects of visual relaxation, making it a powerful tool for mental and physical well-being. A study published in *Frontiers in Psychology* found that as little as 20 minutes spent outdoors can reduce cortisol by up to 21 per cent (PubMed, 2019). This time in nature positively affects our nervous system, bringing us into a restful, parasympathetic state. The impact is even more profound when our focus shifts from a general view to a mindful observation of something specific, such as clouds.

Combining Breathing Exercises with Cloud Gazing

A powerful addition to cloud gazing is to integrate slow, deep breathing. Studies show that deep breathing activates the vagus nerve, a critical component in the PNS, which lowers heart rate and blood pressure (*Journal of Alternative and Complementary Medicine*). As you observe the clouds, take slow, deep breaths, allowing the gentle rhythm of your breath to synchronize with the movement of the clouds. This combination can amplify the calming effect and enhance relaxation.

To make cloud gazing a regular practice, try setting aside a few minutes each day simply to observe the sky. Here's a step-by-step guide:

1. **Find a comfortable spot:** Choose an outdoor spot where you can lie down or sit back comfortably.
2. **Settle into your breath:** Close your eyes for a moment and take a few deep breaths, signalling your body to relax.
3. **Observe without judgement:** Open your eyes, gaze up at the sky and watch the clouds drift by. Notice their shape, size and how they change.

4. **Let thoughts pass by:** As thoughts or emotions arise, imagine them drifting away like clouds, without judgement or attachment.
5. **Finish with gratitude:** Close your eyes again and take a moment to feel grateful for the beauty and calmness of the moment.

Dr Qing Li, a physician and researcher in the field of 'forest bathing', or *shinrin-yoku,* states, 'When we are surrounded by nature, our bodies and minds respond with ease. Sky gazing is an opportunity to immerse in that relaxation, even for a few minutes.'

Dr Andrew Huberman, a neuroscientist, also emphasizes the importance of looking at distant horizons, noting that it stimulates areas of the brain associated with creativity, relaxation and decreased stress. According to Dr Huberman, 'Looking at expansive views, like the sky, can have a potent calming effect on the mind and body.'

Cloud gazing is one of the most accessible tools for mental wellness, offering a natural way to de-stress, practise mindfulness and reconnect with nature. The next time you feel overwhelmed, look up at the sky and let the clouds guide you to a place of peace and clarity.

20

Decluttering Your Space

Have you ever noticed how you feel when you walk into a clean, organized room as opposed to one filled with clutter? That sense of calm you experience in a tidy space is more than just an aesthetic preference; it's a reflection of how our environment affects our nervous system. Clutter doesn't just crowd our physical space—it can create mental chaos, triggering a stress response in our body.

The Accumulation of Clutter: Why We Hoard and Its Hidden Costs

It's easy to accumulate things—clothes, gadgets, papers and trinkets—that we think we might need someday. These items often end up forgotten, collecting dust and taking up space. While buying new things isn't inherently problematic, issues arise when we don't let go of the old to make room for the new. Over time, our drawers, closets and shelves overflow with items that no longer serve a purpose but still demand our attention.

This clutter can be seen as 'dead energy'—objects that no longer contribute to our lives but occupy mental and emotional space. Research shows that living in cluttered environments can lead to feelings of being overwhelmed and contribute to stress. Clutter acts as a constant visual reminder of unfinished tasks and decisions, which can become a source of anxiety, gradually overloading our nervous system. In fact, studies published on PubMed and by NCBI have found that individuals living in disorganized environments often experience higher levels of cortisol, a stress hormone known to activate the sympathetic nervous system.

How Clutter Affects Our Nervous System

The human brain constantly processes information from its environment. In a cluttered space, this influx of visual stimuli creates a form of sensory overload, requiring our brain to work harder to focus on tasks. Our attention becomes scattered, our ability to process information is compromised and we may experience mental fatigue. This phenomenon is supported by research from the Princeton Neuroscience Institute, which found that clutter competes for our attention, reducing performance and increasing stress.

When our surroundings are chaotic, our nervous system can shift into a sympathetic mode, releasing stress hormones that increase alertness, heart rate and muscle tension. Decluttering, on the other hand, allows us to shift back to the parasympathetic mode, promoting relaxation, better focus and overall well-being.

Decluttering is more than just cleaning up; it's a practice of mindfulness that has physical and psychological benefits. Studies reveal that reducing clutter can alleviate symptoms of depression, anxiety and stress, as well as improve mood and cognition. The process of sorting and organizing can also be therapeutic. As we decide which items to keep and which to let go, we engage in reflection, acknowledging the emotional attachments we may have with certain objects. This can help us confront and release past memories, leading to emotional catharsis and growth.

Furthermore, the physical act of decluttering promotes mindful engagement with our environment. By focusing on one task at a time—whether organizing a drawer or clearing off a surface—we create space not only physically but mentally as well. This reduction in sensory input allows our brain to function more optimally, thereby reducing stress and improving our ability to concentrate.

Experts in psychology and neuroscience have noted the powerful effects of decluttering on our mental and emotional well-being. Dr Sherrie Bourg Carter, a psychologist who specializes in stress management, highlights that 'clutter bombards our minds with excessive stimuli, causing our senses to work overtime on stimuli that aren't necessary or important.' This overload, she explains, 'can lead to increased stress and difficulty focusing.' Meanwhile, Dr Darby Saxbe, an expert on home psychology, has pointed out that 'our homes are extensions of ourselves, and a cluttered home can create a cluttered mind, reflecting unresolved issues in our emotional lives.'

Marie Kondo, a well-known organizational consultant, also emphasizes that the process of decluttering can build joy and inner peace. By keeping only the items that 'spark joy', Kondo suggests that we cultivate an environment that reflects our true selves, thus minimizing stress and bringing harmony into our lives.

Environment and Emotion: The Impact of Space on Mood and Behaviour

Our physical surroundings directly affect our emotional states. Studies show that organized environments contribute to positive emotions, while cluttered spaces are linked to negative feelings like frustration, guilt and even depression. This response can be attributed to how our brain interprets our surroundings. A clean, orderly space promotes a sense of control and stability, whereas cluttered spaces often create feelings of chaos and unpredictability.

Imagine stepping into a room filled with disorganized stacks of papers, clothing scattered around and dishes left unwashed. Compare that experience to walking into a clean, organized room where everything has its place. The latter instantly feels more calming and inviting, allowing the nervous system to settle. This soothing effect is not only psychological but physiological as well—an uncluttered environment can help lower blood pressure and slow heart rate, all of which engage the PNS.

Decluttering doesn't have to be an overwhelming task. Start small, with one drawer or a single surface. Consider this an ongoing practice rather than a one-time event. Here are a few tips to help you incorporate mindful decluttering into your life:

1. **Start with a purpose:** Identify why you want to declutter. Are you looking to reduce stress, improve focus or simply create more space for the things you love? Defining a purpose helps make the process intentional.
2. **Work in small steps:** Begin with a manageable area—a drawer, a shelf or your workspace. Small successes build momentum and make larger projects feel achievable.
3. **Sort into categories:** Use categories, like 'keep', 'donate' and 'discard', to streamline your process.
4. **Consider each item's purpose:** Reflect on whether each item serves a current purpose or brings you joy. Letting go of items that no longer serve you can be liberating.
5. **Practise gratitude:** As you declutter, practise gratitude for the items you choose to keep and for the opportunity to create a more peaceful space.
6. **Maintain the routine:** Regularly set aside time to tidy and organize. Decluttering doesn't have to be an exhausting event; it can be a calming routine that brings ongoing peace.

When we let go of things that no longer serve us, we make room for clarity, focus and growth. So, the next time you feel overwhelmed or stuck, look around your space. Decluttering may be the key to unlocking a calmer mind and a more balanced nervous system.

21

Gargling

One surprisingly effective, yet simple, tool to turn on your PNS is gargling. Yes, something as basic as gargling.

At the heart of this lies the vagus nerve. Gargling activates the vagus nerve. When activated, the vagus nerve sends signals to your body to slow down the heart rate, reduce blood pressure and promote relaxation. A higher vagal tone correlates with lower levels of anxiety, depression and stress-related disorders. This is where gargling comes into play as an unexpected, but effective, method for enhancing vagal tone.

The Science Behind Gargling

Gargling involves a repetitive, rhythmic contraction of the muscles in your throat. This activity provides gentle stimulation to the vagus nerve, helping to activate it and thereby promote a parasympathetic response. The action of gargling also stimulates the pharyngeal muscles, which are innervated by the vagus nerve. This stimulation triggers a cascade of physiological responses that encourage relaxation.

A study published in the *Frontiers in Physiology* explored the relationship between vagal nerve stimulation and various health outcomes. The researchers found that activities stimulating the vagus nerve, such as deep breathing and throat muscle contractions (like those involved in gargling), could enhance vagal tone and improve emotional well-being

(Huang et al., 2019). Another study published in the *Frontiers of Physiology* noted that simple throat exercises could lead to significant increases in heart rate variability (HRV), an indicator of improved ANS balance (Patel et al., 2022).

How to Gargle for Maximum Effectiveness

- **Prepare Warm Water:** Fill a glass with warm (not hot) water. Adding a pinch of salt can enhance oral health and provide additional soothing effects.
- **Take a Sip:** Take a mouthful of the warm water but refrain from swallowing it.
- **Tilt Your Head Back:** Slightly tilt your head back to allow the water to reach the back of your throat.
- **Gargle:** Gargle for about 30 seconds, making a continuous 'ahhh' sound. This sound can enhance the stimulation of the vagus nerve.
- **Repeat:** Spit out the water and repeat the process several times, ideally once or twice a day, particularly during stressful moments or before bedtime.

This practice not only promotes relaxation, but also improves oral hygiene, making it a double benefit.

Dr Bessel van der Kolk, a leading trauma researcher, also underscores the significance of body-based interventions in healing trauma and managing stress. He points out that such practices not only ground us but also activate our biological pathways to promote healing.

Gargling, a simple and accessible practice, can help activate the vagus nerve and promote a parasympathetic response, facilitating a transition from stress to relaxation. So, the next time you're feeling stressed or anxious, remember that the answer might just be a glass of warm water away!

22

Salt Lamps

Imagine stepping into a spa. Even before your session begins, a sense of calm washes over you. The soft lighting, the gentle hum of tranquil music and the warm, inviting glow of salt lamps all contribute to this immediate feeling of relaxation. Our environment plays a crucial role in how we feel, and this is the magic we can bring into our own spaces with Himalayan pink salt lamps.

The Science of Himalayan Pink Salt Lamps

Himalayan pink salt lamps are crafted from natural salt crystals sourced from the foothills of the Himalayas. When illuminated, these lamps emit a warm, gentle amber glow that does more than just beautify a room. They are believed to generate negative ions, which can improve air quality and influence the energy of the room.

The Role of Negative Ions

Negative ions are molecules that have gained an electron, making them negatively charged. These ions are naturally found in abundance in places like mountains, forests and near waterfalls. They are thought to have several health benefits, including improving mood, enhancing cognitive function and even alleviating anxiety. According to a study published on *BMC Psychiatry*, exposure to negative ions has been shown to have a positive impact on serotonin levels in the brain, which can help regulate mood and anxiety levels.

Hygroscopic Properties of Salt

The hygroscopic nature of salt means that it attracts and absorbs moisture from the air. This property allows Himalayan pink salt lamps to trap dust, allergens and pollutants, leading to cleaner air and a more comfortable breathing space. A cleaner environment can alleviate symptoms associated with respiratory issues, thereby supporting the transition from a sympathetic nervous system (the fight-or-flight response) to a more relaxed parasympathetic state.

Colour Therapy and the Nervous System

The warm orange hue of the lamp's glow can also be understood through the lens of colour therapy. This particular shade is known for its calming and soothing effects, much like the ambiance of a well-designed spa. According to research, colours can significantly influence our emotional and physiological responses. The soothing qualities of the warm light, emitted by Himalayan salt lamps, may help reduce stress and anxiety, thus promoting relaxation and mindfulness

Personally, I love these lamps and have them lit up almost in every room where I spend the most time. In my office, I keep a Himalayan pink salt lamp on my desk. Its soft glow counteracts the harsh blue light from my computer screen, reducing eye strain and creating a more relaxing work environment.

In my yoga corner, the Himalayan pink salt lamp is a central element. Its warm light enhances the serene atmosphere, making my practice even more soothing. Whether I'm meditating, practising deep breathing or flowing through *asanas*, the lamp's presence deepens my relaxation and connection to the present moment.

In my bedroom, I place a Himalayan pink salt lamp on my bedside table to promote restful sleep. The gentle light creates a tranquil bedtime environment, helping me unwind from the day's activities. As the sun sets and it gets darker, I turn off other lights and let the lamp's light be the only one.

Himalayan pink salt lamps are more than just decorative pieces. We can use something as simple as this to make our environment calmer. Whether in your office, yoga corner or bedroom, these lamps can transform the energy of the room and support a healthier, more relaxed state of being.

Top experts in the field of environmental psychology and holistic wellness have praised Himalayan pink salt lamps for their potential benefits. A study conducted by Hajra Naz and Darakhshan J. Haleem investigated the impact of illuminated salt lamp exposure on serotonin metabolism in rats. The researchers found that prolonged exposure to a salt lamp increased brain tryptophan and serotonin (5-HT) metabolism, suggesting potential antidepressant effects. These findings provide a neurochemical perspective on the claimed benefits of salt lamps.

Research supports the therapeutic benefits attributed to Himalayan pink salt lamps. A study published in the *BMC Psychiatry* journal found that individuals, who spent time in environments enriched with negative ions, reported significant reductions in anxiety and stress levels. These findings reinforce the notion that our surroundings can profoundly influence our psychological and physiological states.

Himalayan pink salt lamps offer a simple, yet effective, tool for enhancing our environments, helping us move from the sympathetic nervous system's stress response to the parasympathetic state of relaxation and rejuvenation.

23

The Half-Salamander

Do you ever feel like your brain might just combust under high stress—anxious thoughts racing, heart pounding, your body in a state of fight-or-flight? It feels overwhelming, but you have more control than you realize. Here's a simple technique to help you switch back to calm mode.

Try the half-salamander exercise. Named after the way your eyes move while your head stays still, much like a salamander, it finds its origin in renowned cranio-sacral therapist, Stanley Rosenberg's book, *Assessing the Healing Power of the Vagus Nerve* (2017).

This simple, yet effective, practice helps you stimulate the vagus nerve, which plays a critical role in your body's ability to relax and recover from stress.

Here's how to do it:

- **Find a comfortable position:** Stand or sit comfortably with your head facing forward.
- **Eye movement:** Look to the right without turning your head.
- **Head tilt:** Slowly tilt your head towards your right shoulder and hold for 30–60 seconds. Focus on deep, calming breaths during this time.
- **Return to neutral:** Gently bring your head back to its neutral position and shift your eyes forward again.

- **Repeat on the other side:** Perform the same steps, this time, looking to the left and tilting your head towards your left shoulder.

The Science Behind It

This exercise works by stimulating the vagus nerve, which helps control your heart rate and triggers a relaxation response in your body. By engaging this nerve, you can help shift your body out of the fight-or-flight mode and into a state of calm and control.

The vagus nerve is the longest cranial nerve in the body and has a significant impact on the ANS, which regulates involuntary bodily functions such as heart rate and digestion. Engaging the vagus nerve can trigger the relaxation response, countering the stress-induced fight-or-flight state.

- A study published in the *American Journal of Physiology*, 'Heart and circulatory physiology', demonstrated that vagus nerve stimulation can decrease heart rate and increase heart rate variability, linked with relaxation and improved health outcomes (Ardell et al., 2015).
- The *Journal of Psychiatric Research* published a study indicating that individuals, who received vagus nerve stimulation, reported significant improvements in anxiety and mood disorders (Grimonprez et al., 2015).

Adding the Half-Salamander to Your Life

The next time you find yourself overwhelmed with stress or anxiety, try the half-salamander exercise. The key is to practise it regularly. Just as you need to strengthen your body through exercise, you can cultivate calmness through intentional practices for the mind.

24
Limiting Caffeine Intake

Caffeine is a ubiquitous part of life for most of us. From that first sip of morning coffee to afternoon tea or energy drinks, many of us rely on this stimulant to enhance alertness and energy. While caffeine has scientifically recognized benefits, its overconsumption can lead to significant negative effects on our nervous system and overall well-being.

The Science of Caffeine

Caffeine is classified as a psychoactive substance and a neuro exciter, meaning, it stimulates the nervous system. It primarily works by blocking adenosine receptors in the brain, which prevents drowsiness and increases wakefulness. This mechanism, while effective for short-term alertness, comes with physiological responses that can negatively affect our nervous system.

When caffeine enters the bloodstream, it triggers the release of hormones like adrenaline and cortisol, which prepare the body for a fight-or-flight response. This hormonal surge increases heart rate, blood pressure and energy levels, providing a temporary boost. However, this is often followed by a crash, leading to feelings of fatigue and sluggishness—a phenomenon commonly referred to as the 'caffeine crash'.

Hormonal Response: Adrenaline and Cortisol

Excessive caffeine intake can keep the body in a state of heightened alertness, leading to chronic stress and anxiety. Research indicates that chronic caffeine consumption can result in over-activation of the adrenal glands, potentially leading to adrenal fatigue. In this state, the glands may fail to produce adequate hormone levels, causing persistent fatigue and other health issues (Schmitt et al., 2015).

Effects on Sleep and Stress

Caffeine significantly interferes with sleep patterns, especially when consumed later in the day. Research published in the *Journal of Clinical Sleep Medicine* found that caffeine intake, even 6 hours before bedtime, could disrupt sleep architecture, making it difficult to fall asleep and achieve restorative sleep (Hirshkowitz et al., 2015). Poor sleep quality exacerbates stress, creating a vicious cycle of reliance on caffeine for energy.

Cortisol levels are naturally higher in the morning to help us wake up. However, consuming caffeine immediately can lead to unnecessary spikes in cortisol, which stresses the body further (López et al., 2018). A study published in *Psychosomatic Medicine* indicated that excessive caffeine could amplify the stress response, leading to increased anxiety and a lower tolerance for stressors (Jansen et al., 2014).

Long-Term Implications of High Caffeine Intake

Chronic high caffeine consumption has been associated with various health issues, including an increased risk of cardiovascular disease. A meta-analysis in *Circulation* concluded that while moderate coffee consumption may offer protective cardiovascular effects, excessive intake could elevate blood pressure and heart rate, contributing to long-term cardiovascular risks (Zhang et al., 2011).

Moreover, studies have shown a correlation between high caffeine intake and anxiety disorders. A study in the *American*

Journal of Psychiatry found that individuals consuming more than 400 mg of caffeine per day exhibited higher levels of anxiety symptoms (Lindgren et al., 2017). This reinforces the importance of limiting caffeine for those prone to stress or anxiety.

Leading food scientists have weighed in on the effects of caffeine as well. Dr William Li, a prominent researcher and author of *Eat to Beat Disease*, emphasizes that while moderate coffee consumption can have health benefits—such as antioxidant properties and improved cognitive function—overconsumption can hinder stress management and overall health. He points out that caffeine's role in stimulating the central nervous system can lead to elevated stress levels, particularly when consumed in excess or at inappropriate times.

According to Dr Li, the key lies in balance: 'Moderation is essential. It's important to recognize how our body reacts to caffeine, particularly if we are experiencing stress or sleep deprivation. This awareness can guide better choices that enhance our health rather than detract from it.'

Moderation is the Key

While moderate caffeine consumption can provide cognitive benefits and improve mood, moderation is key. Scientific studies suggest that consuming 1–2 cups of high-quality coffee per day can be beneficial, as moderate coffee consumption may reduce the risk of certain diseases and enhance cognitive function (Santos et al., 2020). However, problems arise when caffeine consumption exceeds this threshold or is poorly timed.

To reap the most out of your cup of coffee, consider the following guidelines:

1. **Timing is Crucial:** Wait 90 minutes to 2 hours after waking to have your first cup of coffee. This timing allows for a natural increase in cortisol levels without additional stimulation.

2. **Limit Late-Day Intake:** Avoid caffeine consumption in the late afternoon and evening to prevent sleep disturbances.
3. **Monitor Your Body's Signals:** If you experience jitters, anxiety or trouble sleeping, consider reducing your caffeine intake.
4. **Explore Alternatives:** Matcha tea offers a gentler caffeine boost due to its lower caffeine content and the presence of L-theanine, which promotes relaxation without drowsiness.

As someone who enjoys a good cup of coffee, I understand the joy it brings. However, I recognize that not all coffee is created equal. A bad cup can be as disappointing as poorly cooked food. I prioritize quality and always seek out high-quality beans and proper brewing methods.

While I cherish the scientific benefits of my daily cup, I remain mindful of my body's needs. If I find myself sleep-deprived or jet-lagged, I consciously choose to forgo caffeine to prevent adding to my cortisol burden.

Caffeine can be both a friend and a foe. While it offers benefits, such as enhanced alertness and mood improvement, its overconsumption can lead to significant negative effects on the nervous system and stress levels. Use caffeine wisely, and let it serve you—not the other way round.

25

Sitting in Silence

Imagine a world without notifications, without the constant buzz of chatter, news updates and digital pings. Imagine sitting quietly, hearing nothing but the gentle sound of your own breath. In today's overstimulated world, silence has become almost mythical—rare, fleeting and often uncomfortable. We've grown so accustomed to filling every free moment with activity that the idea of simply 'doing nothing' feels foreign. Yet, research shows that the most powerful thing we can do for our well-being might just be sitting in stillness.

Silence isn't simply the absence of noise. It's a return to our natural state of calm, a chance for our nervous system to reset and heal. By simply allowing ourselves moments of quiet, we invite a profound shift in our body. This stillness calms the SNS, which drives our stress responses, and activates the PNS, responsible for rest and recovery. When we enter this state, we aren't just 'relaxing'; we're actually giving our bodies the break they desperately need to repair, restore and rejuvenate.

The Science of Silence

Research has shown that silence, even for short periods, helps regulate the SNS and activate the PNS. In doing so, silence becomes a simple, natural way to bring our nervous system back into balance.

Science has recently begun to uncover how silence affects our body at a physiological level. Here's what studies are finding:

1. **Reduced Cortisol Levels:** Cortisol, the body's primary stress hormone, is released when we're under pressure. Elevated cortisol can have harmful effects on mood, sleep and immunity health. A study in the *Journal of Psychosomatic Research* found that brief periods of silence reduced cortisol levels significantly, helping to mitigate the effects of chronic stress.
2. **Heart Rate Variability (HRV):** HRV is a measure of the variation in time between heartbeats, and it reflects how well the body adapts to stress. Higher HRV is associated with resilience and balanced nervous system function. Research in *Frontiers in Neuroscience* found that regular silence practices improved HRV, suggesting a stronger, more adaptive response to stress.
3. **Increased Neurogenesis:** Remarkably, silence has been shown to encourage the formation of new brain cells. A 2013 study published in *Brain Structure and Function* found that silence led to increased neurogenesis in the hippocampus, a brain region vital for learning, memory and emotional regulation.
4. **Better Sleep Quality:** Silent practices have been linked to improved sleep. Research published in *Applied Psychophysiology and Biofeedback* showed that a daily silence practice led to deeper, more restful sleep, helping individuals recover more effectively from daily stress.

Dr Herbert Benson, known for his groundbreaking research on the relaxation response, emphasizes silence as a pathway to healing. His work shows that relaxation practices, including silence and meditation, activate the PNS, bringing down blood pressure, reducing anxiety and improving overall health.

Harvard neuroscientist Dr Sara Lazar's research echoes this, finding that regular silent practices can even lead to structural changes in the brain, such as increased cortical thickness in areas related to attention, memory and emotion regulation.

Practitioners of Vipassana meditation—a practice based on silent, mindful observation—have long believed in silence as a way to enhance self-awareness and emotional balance. Through Vipassana, individuals learn to observe thoughts and feelings without judgement, which calms the nervous system and improves mental clarity. Silence, they suggest, is not just a practice; it's a teacher that reveals the mind's natural state of balance.

Starting Your Practice of Silence

The beauty of silence is that it's accessible to everyone. All you need is a few minutes each day, a quiet spot and the willingness to simply be still. Here's a practical guide to get you started:

1. **Choose Your Quiet Space:** Find a place where you won't be disturbed, even if it's just a comfortable chair in a quiet corner. Silence doesn't require absolute stillness, only fewer distractions.
2. **Set a Timer:** Start with 5 minutes, gradually working your way up. A timer will help you relax, knowing you're setting aside this time without constantly checking the clock.
3. **Anchor in Your Breath:** Begin by observing your breathing. Notice each inhale and exhale. Feel the stillness in the brief pause at the end of each breath.
4. **Engage the Five Senses:** Gradually tune into your senses:
    - **Taste:** Notice any taste in your mouth, or think of a comforting flavour.
    - **Touch:** Feel your hands resting on your lap, or place a hand over your heart to feel its rhythm.
    - **Smell:** Take note of any scents around you.

- **Sight:** If you're sitting with your eyes open, softly gaze at something in front of you.
- **Sound:** Listen to any background noise, eventually finding the quiet within.

5. **Let Thoughts Pass:** Your mind will wander—this is natural. Acknowledge each thought without judgement, and gently bring your focus back to your breath or senses.

Finding Silence in Everyday Life

Silence can be an antidote to the stress of daily life. Rather than reaching for coffee, scrolling through social media or tuning into another podcast, give yourself the gift of stillness. If you're feeling particularly stressed, try sitting in silence for 10 minutes. During this time, you'll begin to notice a calming shift within. When you return to your day, you'll do so with a clearer, more grounded mind.

For those who find silence challenging at bedtime, this can be an excellent opportunity to unwind. Practise sitting in silence before you sleep, allowing thoughts from the day to settle. You'll likely find your sleep quality improve as your nervous system gets a chance to down-regulate.

Over the last few months, I've started to appreciate the profound peace that comes from silence. Each morning, I sit in quiet reflection, observing my breath, noticing the subtle sounds around me and feeling the stillness. I've discovered something truly beautiful: thoughts, emotions and even life's noise all rise from a place of stillness and return there. This pattern reminds me that peace is always within reach, no matter the turmoil around me.

Practising silence has given me a new way to approach life's challenges. I notice how, even in anger or frustration, there's a quiet underneath, a stable ground I can always come back to. This practice has become my way of returning to balance, day after day. I invite you to try it yourself—to see if even a few moments of silence each day can bring a greater sense of peace to your life.

26

Warm Bath/Feet Soaking (Epsom Salt Baths)

Imagine sinking into a warm bath after a long, demanding day—the heat loosens your tight muscles, the gentle water relaxes you and your mind, almost instinctively, begins to slow down. In that moment, you're not just indulging in a comforting ritual; you're actively supporting one of the most powerful systems in your body: your nervous system.

A warm bath or foot soak, especially when enhanced with Epsom salt, is a simple, yet scientifically grounded, way to encourage your body to shift from a state of 'fight-or-flight' to a state of 'rest-and-digest'. Studies published on PubMed and other research platforms consistently show that warm baths and Epsom salt soaks are far more than just self-care luxuries; they are valuable tools for managing stress, reducing inflammation, enhancing recovery and supporting our overall well-being.

The Science of Warm Baths

When you immerse yourself in warm water, the gentle heat raises your body temperature, prompting blood vessels to dilate and circulation to improve. This increase in blood flow helps ease tight, sore muscles and leads to a cascade of calming effects on the body. The thermoreceptors on your skin sense the heat and relay signals directly to the vagus nerve. This nerve plays a key role in switching off the stress response, telling your body that it's safe to relax.

Studies have shown that warm baths can trigger what's known as the 'relaxation response', discovered by Dr Herbert Benson at Harvard Medical School. This response counteracts the stress-induced 'fight-or-flight' state by slowing heart rate, lowering blood pressure and reducing levels of cortisol and adrenaline—our primary stress hormones. According to research, the warmth from a bath can also improve mood by promoting serotonin release, a neurotransmitter that contributes to feelings of well-being and happiness.

Epsom Salt: Why Magnesium Matters

The benefits of warm baths can be elevated with the addition of Epsom salt, a naturally occurring mineral compound, also known as magnesium sulphate. Magnesium is crucial for over 300 biochemical reactions in the body, including those related to nerve function and muscle relaxation. When we're under chronic stress, our bodies rapidly deplete magnesium stores, which can lead to muscle tension, irritability and an increased stress response.

Topical magnesium absorption, through Epsom salt baths, is a widely accepted method for replenishing this essential mineral. Research indicates that magnesium can be absorbed through the skin, particularly when dissolved in warm water. Once absorbed, magnesium has a calming effect on the nervous system, promoting gamma-aminobutyric acid (GABA) production—a neurotransmitter that slows neural activity and allows the mind to enter a state of relaxation.

Dr Robert Rountree, an integrative medicine physician, explains that 'magnesium is often called the "original chill pill" because of its calming effects on the nervous system'. He goes on to say, 'An Epsom salt bath is one of the best ways to restore magnesium, especially for people dealing with stress or physical exhaustion. It's a great, gentle way to help the body relax.'

Researchers have found that practices promoting parasympathetic activity, like warm baths, had substantial impacts on reducing stress and improving mood and cognitive performance. Regularly engaging in this type of relaxation practice can make the body more resilient to future stressors and create a state of calm and clarity.

Practical Tips: Optimizing Your Bath for Maximum Benefits

1. **Set the Ideal Temperature:** Warm water between 92°F –100°F (33°C–38°C) is best. This range is soothing without causing overheating, which can disrupt relaxation.
2. **Epsom Salt Dosage:** Aim for two cups of Epsom salt in a standard bathtub. This concentration is optimal for magnesium absorption and delivers therapeutic effects.
3. **Soak Duration:** Allow yourself 15–20 minutes to unwind fully, as this duration helps your muscles relax and allows time for magnesium absorption.
4. **Stay Hydrated:** Keep a glass of water nearby, as warm baths can lead to dehydration if you soak for extended periods.
5. **Enhance with Essential Oils:** A few drops of lavender or eucalyptus essential oils can further enhance relaxation. These oils have calming properties that, combined with the bath, create a multi-sensory experience for unwinding.
6. **Foot Soaks on the Go:** For frequent travellers, carrying sachets of Epsom salt in your luggage can make a hotel room feel like a sanctuary. A warm foot soak can be just as effective in calming your nervous system and helping you sleep better on the road.

Incorporating warm baths and Epsom salt soaks into your life is more than a relaxing ritual—it's a scientifically backed method to support your nervous system, enhance stress resilience and promote a state of mental and physical relaxation. From home to hotel, these practices allow you to create moments of calm and rejuvenation, providing your body and mind with the restoration they need to thrive.

27

Limiting Multitasking

In today's world, many of us wear 'multitasking' like a badge of honour. We juggle deadlines at work, navigate busy social calendars, respond to a never-ending stream of emails and manage our personal lives—all while checking our phones every few minutes.

While it seems like multitasking could help us get more done, the reality is far from it. Our brains are not built to handle multiple tasks at once, especially in the way our fast-paced culture demands. And while we may think we're being productive, research has shown that multitasking often does more harm than good, both to our productivity and, crucially, to our nervous system.

Multitasking, in reality, is less about doing several things at once and more about task-switching—rapidly shifting focus from one task to another. This might seem efficient, but this constant redirection of attention strains our brain, draining its energy, heightening stress and leading to mental fatigue. In fact, neuroscience has revealed that multitasking is a significant driver of chronic stress, which, in turn, keeps us locked in the sympathetic 'fight-or-flight' mode.

The result? Increased anxiety, heightened irritability, decreased attention and a risk of burnout.

Science suggests that by moving away from multitasking and learning to focus on one task at a time, we can support a healthier balance between our SNS and PNS. Not only does this approach reduce stress, but it also enhances productivity and emotional well-being.

Why Our Brains Struggle to Do It All

The myth of multitasking stems from a misunderstanding of how our brains process information. Unlike computers that can simultaneously handle multiple processes, our brains can only focus on one complex task at a time. This is due to how our prefrontal cortex, the brain's command centre, handles cognitive tasks.

When we try to multitask, we engage in what researchers call 'task-switching', which is not the same as handling tasks simultaneously. Task-switching involves rapidly moving attention between tasks, which disrupts the brain's natural flow and creates what neuroscientists call 'switch costs'. These are the cognitive 'penalties' that we pay each time we interrupt a task to focus on something else, such as increased error rates, slower reaction times and impaired working memory.

A study from the University of London demonstrated that multitasking lowers IQ scores, similar to losing a night's sleep. The cognitive load of constantly shifting between tasks overloads our brain's processing capacity, which can create mental fatigue and reduce overall effectiveness. In short, what feels like productivity is actually the opposite—each switch between tasks depletes mental resources and limits our cognitive bandwidth.

Multitasking and the Nervous System: The Impact on Stress and Well-Being

When we engage in multitasking, especially with high-pressure deadlines or multiple digital distractions, our brain triggers a stress response, activating the SNS.

This constant activation of the SNS raises cortisol levels, the body's primary stress hormone. Chronically high cortisol levels have been linked to issues like anxiety, depression, poor immune function and even memory impairment. What's worse, when we're locked into this stress state, our ability to tap into the PNS mode diminishes.

By minimizing multitasking, we can help regulate our nervous system and shift from a stressed, 'fight-or-flight' state to a calm, 'rest-and-digest' state. Focusing on one task at a time lowers mental strain and reduces the need for frequent stress responses, allowing the body to rely more on the parasympathetic system.

Research published in the *Journal of Experimental Psychology* highlighted how those who limited task-switching experienced lower stress levels and greater mental clarity. By committing to single-tasking, individuals can sustain focus for longer periods and engage more deeply with tasks. This deep focus not only reduces errors and enhances productivity but also promotes mental relaxation. In this way, we're supporting a more balanced nervous system and gradually retraining our body to exit the constant state of arousal typical of chronic multitaskers.

Furthermore, practising single-tasking has a lasting impact on brain function. Neuroplasticity studies show that by repeatedly engaging in focused work, without distraction, we can retrain the brain, strengthening pathways that support concentration, self-control and emotional regulation. This is important for long-term stress resilience, as a well-regulated brain and nervous system are better equipped to handle daily challenges without feeling overwhelmed.

The Power of Deep Work and Flow States

Enter the concept of 'deep work'—a term coined by Cal Newport, a professor and productivity expert. Deep work involves immersing oneself in a task for a dedicated period, minimizing or eliminating distractions. Newport argues that by engaging in deep work, we can achieve a state of flow—a heightened state of focus where we lose track of time and become fully absorbed in our task.

Flow states have been shown to activate the PNS, promoting relaxation, while simultaneously enhancing creativity and problem-solving abilities. A study conducted by psychologist Mihaly Csikszentmihalyi found that people experience increased happiness and reduced stress when they engage in tasks that demand their full attention and challenge them. This aligns with findings that deep work leads to better mental health, as it allows us to accomplish more meaningful work without the stress-inducing effects of multitasking.

Practical Tips for Limiting Multitasking and Embracing Deep Focus

1. **Designate Focused Time Blocks:** Set aside 1–2 hours for deep work without any distractions. This dedicated time allows your brain to adjust to a single task and supports the PNS.
2. **Use the Pomodoro Technique:** Work for 25 minutes on a single task, then take a 5-minute break. This method helps build focus while providing breaks that prevent mental fatigue.
3. **Turn off Notifications:** Our phones and laptops are constant sources of distraction. Disable notifications to prevent unnecessary interruptions and maintain your focus.
4. **Engage in Mindful Breaks:** Mindful activities, such as deep breathing, meditation or a quick walk, activate the PNS, helping to relieve stress and promote relaxation.
5. **Prioritize Tasks with Purpose:** By organizing tasks based on importance and relevance, you can focus on fewer tasks and dedicate your energy to what matters most, reducing the urge to multitask.

Dr Sandra Chapman, founder of the Center for BrainHealth at the University of Texas, Dallas, emphasizes that the brain's productivity 'tanks' when we multitask, leading to mental fatigue and increased stress. Similarly, Dr Earl Miller, a neuroscientist at MIT, states that multitasking is 'not possible for the human brain'. According to Dr Miller, every time we switch between tasks, we're forcing our brain to recalibrate, which is exhausting and ineffective.

The science is clear: multitasking doesn't make us more productive; it makes us stressed, less efficient and more prone to errors. In a world that celebrates busyness, the choice to focus on one thing at a time is a powerful way to protect and nurture our mental and physical health.

28

Mindful Breathing Breaks/Unplanned Pauses

Picture this: it's 3 p.m. on a Wednesday, and you're buried under a mountain of deadlines. Your to-do list seems to grow longer by the minute, and you can feel the tension creeping into your shoulders. You glance at the clock, wishing for just a moment of relief.

In our whirlwind lives, where busyness is often celebrated, the thought of taking a break can feel like a crime against productivity. Yet, what if I told you that stepping away from your work—even for a minute—could be one of the most powerful gifts you give yourself?

Imagine pausing to take a few deep breaths, letting go of that tightness in your chest, and emerging from that brief interlude with clarity and renewed energy. This is the magic of mindful breathing breaks—simple, unplanned pauses that can help you reconnect with yourself and regulate your nervous system.

When we dive headfirst into our work, our SNS gets activated, triggering a cascade of stress responses that leave us feeling drained. However, here's the good news: taking mindful breaks allows us to activate our PNS, inviting a sense of calm and restoring balance.

However, not all breaks are created equal. It's easy to fall into the trap of scrolling through social media or binge-watching videos as a way to unwind, thinking we're taking a break. Yet, these activities often leave us feeling more overwhelmed and disconnected. On the other hand, using our breaks for activities that truly nourish our mind and body—like listening to music, doing a few stretches or engaging in mindful breathing—can turn a moment of downtime into a powerful opportunity for renewal.

The Power of Mindful Breathing Breaks

Whether you're in the midst of a busy workday or navigating the demands of everyday life, remember that a moment of mindful breathing can be your secret weapon for resilience and clarity.

Research has consistently shown that mindful breathing can effectively stimulate the PNS and counteract the stress-induced effects of the SNS. A study by Jerath et al. (2006) highlights how deep breathing techniques can enhance heart rate variability—a key indicator of the body's ability to respond to stress.

One-Minute Breathing Exercise

Let's try a simple mindful breathing exercise that takes only a minute but can have a significant impact:

1. Find a quiet, comfortable place to sit, with your back straight.
2. Close your eyes and take in a deep breath through your nose, filling your lungs completely.
3. Hold your breath till the count of four.
4. Slowly, exhale through your mouth, emptying your lungs completely.
5. Repeat this cycle for one minute, focusing only on your breath.
6. If your mind wanders (which it likely will!), gently acknowledge the thought and bring your attention back to your breath.

While you practise this technique:

- Feel the sensation of your breath moving in and out of your body.
- Pay attention to how your chest or belly rises and falls.
- Avoid trying to control your breathing; just observe it.

By concentrating on your breath, you cultivate mindfulness and presence. The goal isn't to achieve a specific state but to simply be in this moment. When you finish, you can return to your tasks with a clearer mind and a more relaxed body.

Ideas for Taking Breaks

To make the most of your breaks, consider incorporating a variety of activities that promote relaxation and rejuvenation. Here are some effective ways to take mindful breaks:

- **Listen to music:** Play a favourite song or soothing instrumental track to uplift your mood.
- **Stretch or do yoga:** Perform a few simple stretches or yoga poses to release physical tension.
- **Practise breathing exercises:** Spend a few minutes focusing on deep, mindful breathing to reset your nervous system.
- **Hydrate:** Drink a glass of water to refresh and rehydrate your body.
- **Take a short walk:** Step outside for a brief walk to get some fresh air and a change of scenery.
- **Meditate:** Use a few minutes to meditate and clear your mind, even if just for a moment.
- **Journal:** Write down your thoughts or make a list of things you're grateful for to help shift your perspective.
- **Read a book:** Spend a few minutes reading a few pages of a book or a meaningful article that interests you.
- **Practise visualization:** Close your eyes and visualize a peaceful scene, like a beach or a forest, to transport your mind to a calming place.

- **Enjoy a healthy snack:** Refuel your body with a nutritious snack to boost your energy and mood.
- **Connect with a friend:** Have a quick chat with a friend or colleague to share a laugh or catch up on life.
- **Observe nature:** If possible, spend a few moments observing nature, whether it's watching the clouds, tending to a plant or enjoying a view.
- **Just BE:** Allow yourself to do nothing for a moment—just sit in silence and be present.

The Importance of Mindful Breaks

Taking breaks thoughtfully can be a powerful tool for regulating our nervous system. It doesn't have to be an elaborate or lengthy pause to be effective. Sometimes, even a brief 2-minute break can be incredibly revitalizing.

The next time you feel the pressure to push through without pause, consider making it a moment of mindfulness instead. You might find that you return to your tasks feeling more refreshed, focused and ready to face whatever comes your way.

29

Stargazing

Life often feels like a race we didn't sign up for. Between endless to-do's, constant notifications and the hustle of everyday demands, finding a moment of peace can seem impossible. Yet, one of the most powerful ways to unwind is also one of the simplest: just looking up. There's a quiet magic in lying under a starlit sky, a sense of comfort that reminds us how small our daily worries really are. As we take in the vastness above, we're reminded that life is bigger than our stress, and that sometimes, all we need to do is pause.

Whether lying on a beach, reclining on a forest floor or simply stepping outside your front door on a clear night, stargazing has a remarkable ability to tap into our body's natural mechanisms for relaxation. But what is it about this activity that has such a calming effect, and how does it actually work within our nervous system?

How Stargazing Shifts the Nervous System

When we lie back, gaze up and let our minds wander across the stars, a cascade of changes begins within our body and brain. Our heart rate decreases, breathing slows and muscles relax. Scientifically, stargazing creates a calming response similar to other forms of nature immersion, which are increasingly recognized for their ability to reduce stress hormones and encourage parasympathetic activation.

The Science Behind Stargazing and Nervous System Regulation

1. **Awe and Perspective**
   The sense of awe is a powerful emotional state that has been linked to numerous mental and physical benefits. According to studies published in *Frontiers in Psychology*, experiences of awe—whether inspired by nature, art or vastness, like a star-filled sky—have been shown to reduce inflammatory markers and lower stress. Researchers argue that awe, which often involves a feeling of 'being part of something bigger', reduces self-focused rumination and activates a parasympathetic response, calming the nervous system and reducing heart rate and blood pressure. Dr Dacher Keltner, a psychologist at UC Berkeley, describes awe as an 'antidote to anxiety', noting that it helps people feel smaller in the best way possible, decreasing their perceived burdens and worries. Stargazing, by inspiring awe, taps into this natural stress-relief mechanism, shifting focus away from personal concerns to the grand scale of the cosmos.
2. **Mindfulness and Reduced Mental Noise**
   Stargazing also engages the brain in a natural form of mindfulness. Studies in *Journal of Psychiatric Research* suggests that mindfulness practices have a profound effect on the nervous system, lowering cortisol levels and increasing heart rate variability (a marker of parasympathetic activation). When we stargaze, we naturally become present, quieting the brain's ongoing cycle of stress-related thoughts. This relaxed, mindful state can create a significant drop in the activity of the amygdala, the brain region responsible for detecting threats and sparking the fight-or-flight response.

3. **Engagement of the Relaxation Response**
   The concept of the 'relaxation response', first introduced by Dr Herbert Benson of Harvard Medical School, is a physical state that can be achieved through practices such as deep breathing, meditation and nature exposure. Stargazing aligns with these principles by creating a tranquil, rhythmic breathing pattern as we relax and focus on the stars. This process stimulates the vagus nerve, an essential nerve in the PNS. The vagus nerve's activation helps reduce the heart rate and promotes a calm, restorative state in the body.

Experts on stress and nature therapy continue to support the idea that nature engagement, including stargazing, provides unique benefits for mental and physical health. Dr Qing Li, an expert on 'forest bathing', believes that the effects extend to all natural settings. According to his research, 'nature exposure is a powerful tool that can promote relaxation, reduce anxiety and decrease sympathetic nervous activity.'

In Japan, studies on *shinrin-yoku* (forest bathing) have demonstrated significant reductions in cortisol levels and improvements in mood after participants simply spent time in natural environments. Stargazing, as a specific form of nature exposure, invites a similarly calming response, helping to transition the nervous system into a state of rest.

Dr Lisa Nisbet, a psychologist specializing in nature and mental health, notes, 'Our brain craves a natural environment for restoration.' She describes how even brief periods of exposure to natural settings can have a lasting impact on our nervous system and mental well-being. In her view, stargazing taps into this innate need for natural immersion, where the vastness of the universe plays a profound role in reducing our mental load.

For those seeking an accessible way to regulate their nervous system and find peace, stargazing requires no special training or complex set-up. It's an open invitation to simply look up.

Here are some practical tips:

1. **Find a dark, quiet place:** Light pollution can diminish the visibility of stars, so aim for areas outside city limits, a local park or even a designated dark-sky location, if available.
2. **Leave your phone behind:** Let this experience be free of distractions. If you use an app to find constellations, try switching it off after orientation so you can be present.
3. **Engage in rhythmic breathing:** Deep, slow breathing, while gazing at the stars, encourages parasympathetic activation, enhancing the relaxation effects of stargazing.
4. **Add a guided meditation (optional):** For those who want a bit more guidance, consider using a nature-based meditation app that can pair well with stargazing. This helps to keep your mind focused on the present moment.
5. **Embrace a sense of wonder:** Let your mind drift, and welcome any thoughts or emotions that arise. Research suggests that simply embracing awe, as you stargaze, can amplify the calming effects.

Stargazing, the ancient practice of looking to the heavens, is as scientifically significant as it is nourishing for the soul. By encouraging our body's natural parasympathetic responses and helping to downregulate stress, it offers a deeply accessible form of self-care. The simple act of lying beneath the stars, surrounded by the quiet of the night, is one of the most profound ways we can tap into our nervous system's innate ability to rest and restore.

30

Engaging in Artistic Expression

Art is more than just a pastime; it is a powerful avenue for self-expression that allows individuals to process emotions. Activities like drawing, painting, colouring and doodling serve as vital tools for down-regulating an upregulated nervous system, easing stress and creating a peaceful state of mind. Through colours, shapes and forms, we externalize our internal states, capturing emotions that often elude verbal expression. No, one does not have to be a Picasso to paint!

Art used as a means to express can't be graded; it is about how one feels. In traditional art education, the emphasis on judgement can lead to feelings of reluctance to explore this beautiful form of self-healing. However, when art is approached as a form of personal expression, free from judgement, it opens the door to a powerful emotional release and healing.

I had the privilege of witnessing this transformative power of art, first-hand, during my visit at a de-addiction centre in Switzerland. I met an inspiring art therapist who introduced me to artistic expression in a way I had never imagined. Unlike my previous experiences in school, where our creations were subject to evaluation, this session allowed me to explore drawing, painting and colouring without any expectations. With a soothing piano playlist in the background, I immersed myself in the experience, discovering the joy of simply playing with colours.

This liberating session illuminated the therapeutic potential of art for many individuals, including my patients, who seek joy, peace and a means of expression. It reinforced the idea that art therapy is invaluable for those facing substance use disorders, behavioural addictions, burnout and even those simply searching for new paths in life.

Artistic expression encompasses a wide range of activities, each offering unique therapeutic benefits:

- **Drawing and Painting:** These activities allow individuals to communicate their emotions through colour and form. Research indicates that engaging in these practices can lead to improved emotional well-being and reduced anxiety.
- **Pottery:** The tactile nature of pottery provides grounding experiences that help individuals connect with their senses. This connection promotes mindfulness, thus encouraging relaxation and emotional regulation.
- **Crafting:** Engaging in crafting activities builds a sense of accomplishment and joy. Research published in the *Journal of Positive Psychology* suggests that engaging in creative activities boosts mood and enhances overall well-being.
- **Doodling:** Often underestimated, doodling encourages relaxation and mindfulness. It allows the mind to wander freely, promoting a flow state that reduces stress and enhances focus.

Numerous studies support the assertion that art serves as an effective medium for emotional expression and stress reduction:

- **Cortisol Reduction:** Dr Girija Kaimal's research indicates that engaging in art-making for just 45 minutes can significantly lower cortisol levels, a key stress hormone. It highlights art's potential as a simple yet effective stress management tool (Kaimal et al., 2016).

- **Mindfulness and Concentration:** Adult colouring books and mandala art have gained popularity for their calming effects. Research shows that these structured activities induce mindfulness, helping participants focus and enhance concentration. A study published in *Psychology of Aesthetics, Creativity, and the Arts* found that colouring mandalas promoted a state of relaxation and mindfulness among participants.
- **Emotional Regulation:** Engaging with art activates regions of the brain involved in emotion regulation, such as the limbic system. This activation facilitates emotional processing and can be particularly beneficial for trauma survivors, as indicated by research in the *International Journal of Art Therapy*.

Art therapy isn't limited to a single demographic; it benefits all ages, from children to older adults. Each group finds unique therapeutic and emotional value in creative expression:

- **Children:** Art provides a natural outlet for children to express emotions they might not yet be able to put into words. Young children often find it challenging to articulate their emotions verbally, but through drawing and colouring, they gain a tangible way to explore their feelings. Research from the *Journal of Pediatric Oncology Nursing* suggests that engaging children in creative activities reduces symptoms of anxiety and enhances emotional resilience, helping them develop healthier coping skills.
- **Teens and Young Adults:** Adolescents often experience high levels of stress and emotional turmoil as they navigate developmental changes. Artistic expression helps teenagers process these feelings, while also promoting self-identity and emotional resilience. Creative arts programmes in schools, for instance, have been shown to lower anxiety and boost self-esteem among adolescents, according to a study

published in *Psychology of Aesthetics, Creativity, and the Arts*.

- **Adults and Seniors:** For adults, art is a way to step out of the daily grind and reconnect with creativity and mindfulness. Many seniors, in particular, benefit from adult colouring books or crafting activities, which can help enhance cognitive function, improve hand–eye coordination and reduce feelings of loneliness and depression. Studies show that art activities can also protect against memory decline, providing a calming way for seniors to engage in mindful, meditative work.

Art therapists provide structured support for individuals working through stress, trauma or mental health challenges. They create a safe, non-judgemental environment, where clients can freely express and explore complex feelings. Art therapy has been especially effective for trauma survivors, as it helps them access non-verbal ways to process experiences that are otherwise difficult to discuss. Findings published by NCBI indicate that visual art therapy significantly improves post-traumatic stress disorder (PTSD) symptoms, reduces anxiety and enhances emotional regulation. This is because art activates both hemispheres of the brain, encouraging holistic emotional integration and promoting deeper self-acceptance.

Whether through painting, colouring, crafting, or any other form of creative activity, art provides a safe and effective means to explore, understand and release our feelings. By engaging in artistic practices, we not only process emotions but also develop mindfulness and concentration, enhancing our overall well-being.

Expression is a crucial aspect of emotional processing and healing. Whether through art, writing, music or another form, finding a way to express our emotions is essential for our mental and emotional health. Artistic expression provides a beautiful and effective channel for this, allowing us to explore, understand and release our feelings in a safe and constructive manner.

31

Restorative Yoga Poses

Yoga has long been recognized for its ability to restore balance to both the body and mind. What makes restorative yoga particularly effective is its gentle approach. Unlike other forms of yoga, that build intensity, restorative yoga encourages relaxation through passive, supported poses held for extended periods.

Restorative yoga focuses on complete relaxation, with each pose fully supported by props like bolsters, blankets and blocks to ensure there is no strain on the body. Both practices are designed to activate the PNS, making them ideal for highly stressed individuals.

Besides the asanas, breath work also plays an integral role in restorative yoga. When we breathe deeply and consciously, through the poses, it sends signals to the brain that the body is safe, thus encouraging a relaxation response. Diaphragmatic breathing, commonly practised in restorative poses, stimulates the vagus nerve, a key player in the PNS.

Here are a few restorative yoga poses that help calm the nervous system and promote deep relaxation:

1. ***Balasana* (Supported Child's Pose)**
   In this pose, the body is draped over a bolster or cushion, allowing the spine to lengthen and the hips to release. Balasana helps calm the mind, relieve tension in the lower back and encourage deep, diaphragmatic

breathing. This pose is especially effective for reducing stress and anxiety, making it a favourite among restorative yoga practitioners.

2. ***Supta Baddha Konasana* (Reclined Bound Angle Pose)**
   In this heart-opening pose, the body is supported with props under the spine, head and knees, allowing the chest to expand gently. This pose encourages relaxation of the chest and shoulders, areas where stress tends to accumulate. It also stimulates the PNS by opening the front body and allowing for deeper, fuller breaths.
3. ***Viparita Karani* (Legs Up the Wall)**
   This gentle inversion is one of the most soothing poses for the nervous system. With the legs resting against the wall and the body fully supported, this pose helps reverse the effects of gravity, promoting blood flow to the heart and brain. It is deeply relaxing and can help reduce anxiety, insomnia and fatigue.
4. ***Supta Matsyendrasana* (Supported Reclining Twist)**
   Twists are known to detoxify the body and release tension in the spine. In a restorative version, the body is fully supported with props, allowing for a gentle, soothing stretch. This pose is excellent for relieving tension in the lower back and calming the mind.
5. ***Savasana* (Corpse Pose)**
   Savasana is the ultimate restorative pose, allowing for full relaxation of the body and mind. By lying in a neutral position, supported by blankets and bolsters, the nervous system can completely relax. This pose is essential for integrating the benefits of the practice, allowing the body to absorb the calming effects of the previous poses.

The impact of restorative yoga on the nervous system has been studied in various scientific settings.

One study published in *Psychoneuroendocrinology* found that yoga, particularly restorative practices, significantly reduced cortisol levels in participants, showing a measurable reduction in stress.

A 2014 study published in *Journal of Clinical Oncology* also demonstrated that restorative yoga could enhance immune function by increasing the activity of natural killer cells, which are essential for protecting the body from infections and illnesses. This suggests that the calming effects of restorative yoga not only benefit the nervous system but also contribute to overall physical health.

Restorative yoga is actually a great outlet for highly stressed individuals to step out of their sympathetic overdrive and into a space of healing and renewal. For those who are constantly on the go, this practice offers an opportunity to reset and recalibrate the nervous system. It teaches the body how to relax again, something many of us have forgotten how to do. By practising restorative yoga regularly, we train the nervous system to shift more easily from the stress of the sympathetic mode into the peace and calm of the parasympathetic mode—even if it just means a 15-minute practice daily, in case one doesn't have time to spend an hour-long session.

32

Visualization and Guided Imagery

Visualization isn't just about daydreaming or wishful thinking—they are scientifically backed methods for down-regulating our nervous system, helping us shift from a state of fight-or-flight to a state of rest and relaxation. It is something we add to every patient's protocol because if our mind can't see it, it becomes very difficult to achieve it.

But what exactly are they, and how do they work?

Visualization is the practice of creating vivid mental images in your mind—imagining yourself in a peaceful setting, achieving a goal or even picturing your body healing itself. Guided imagery takes this a step further, often involving a recorded voice or a coach who leads you through a specific scenario or scene, like walking on a serene beach or sitting by a calm lake. It's like a mental movie where your mind plays out, and the results can be surprisingly powerful.

How Visualization Works: The Brain's Magic

One of the fascinating things about our brains is that they don't always differentiate between what's real and what's imagined. When you picture something vividly, your brain often responds as though it's really happening. Neuroscientific studies have shown that the same areas of the brain activate when you imagine a scenario as when you actually experience it (Kosslyn et al., 2001).

For example, think about a time when a scary thought suddenly crossed your mind—it might have sent a shiver down your spine, quickened your heartbeat or made you feel a little anxious. Conversely, when you picture yourself lying on a tranquil beach with the sound of waves in the background, you may notice a sense of calm wash over you. Yet, nothing has physically changed. You've probably not even moved an inch while reading this, but those mere thoughts led to chemical changes in your body.

Visualization has gained traction not only through scientific research but also through the teachings of influential thinkers like Joe Dispenza and Bruce Lipton. Joe Dispenza, a leading figure in the field of neuroscience and personal transformation, emphasizes the power of the mind to create our reality. He suggests that through visualization, we can retrain our brains to release old patterns and embrace new ways of thinking and being. Dispenza often states that 'the brain doesn't know the difference between the internal world of thoughts and the external world of reality'. By repeatedly visualizing a desired outcome, we begin to rewire our neural pathways, creating new patterns that align with that reality.

Dr Bruce Lipton, a renowned cell biologist, and my mentor, has long explored how our thoughts influence our physical bodies. I have had the privilege of having him on my podcast and spending loads of time learning under him on the beautiful island of the Maldives.

He beautifully talks about how thoughts create chemistry, meaning, what we think directly affects our cellular processes. He believes that when we visualize positive scenarios, we trigger the release of neurotransmitters like serotonin and dopamine, which can improve our mood and support healing.

Visualization and the Subconscious Mind

The power of visualization lies not just in its ability to calm the nervous system but also in how it affects our subconscious mind. Our subconscious mind is like a fertile ground where thoughts, beliefs and images can take root and grow.

Visualization helps to reprogramme our subconscious mind by consistently feeding it positive images and scenarios. Over time, this can lead to a shift in our thoughts, behaviours and even our emotional health.

Guided imagery is often used in therapy and healing practices to help individuals overcome stress, trauma and anxiety. Studies have shown that guided imagery can significantly reduce stress and anxiety levels, enhance well-being and improve quality of life (Lewandowski et al., 2011). For example, a study published on PubMed found that patients who practised guided imagery before surgery reported lower anxiety levels and a faster recovery rate post-surgery, compared to those who didn't engage in the practice.

Why Visualization Is Challenging for Some People

While visualization has a lot of potential, it's not always easy for everyone. Many people struggle with it due to common obstacles like fear, lack of self-worth or not having a clear vision. When you're bogged down by doubts or are overly critical of yourself, it can be hard to see yourself thriving, achieving goals or being in a place of peace. Others might not have faith in the process, feeling that imagining something couldn't possibly change their reality.

One key to overcoming these obstacles is to start small—visualize a simple scene that makes you happy or calm, like your favourite place in nature or a moment where you felt truly at peace. Over time, as you build trust in the practice, you can start exploring more detailed visualizations, like imagining yourself achieving a personal goal or overcoming a challenge.

Visualization in Action: An Example

Let's try a simple exercise right now.

Imagine you're sitting on a warm, sunlit beach.

You can hear the gentle waves lapping against the shore.

The sun feels warm on your skin, and a cool breeze brushes across your face.

You take in a deep breath, and as you exhale, you feel all your tension melting away into the sand beneath you.

What did you notice?

Simply reading those words, your body might have responded to the imagery. Maybe your shoulders relaxed a bit, or you took a deeper breath. This is the magic of visualization at work, turning thoughts into physical sensations.

The Science Behind Visualization

There's a growing body of research highlighting the effects of visualization on the nervous system. A study published by NCBI found that guided imagery significantly lowered cortisol levels—a key stress hormone—in patients, helping them transition into a more relaxed state (Menzies et al., 2014).

Another study on PubMed revealed that using guided imagery can lead to improvements in sleep quality and reduce symptoms of anxiety and depression in participants (Jallo et al., 2014).

Visualization is also used by athletes as part of mental training. Imagining themselves performing their sport successfully can enhance motor skills and performance. The same brain regions light up during mental practice as during physical practice, showing that visualization can help the brain 'rehearse' tasks, making them easier to perform in reality (Guillot and Collet, 2005). Since our brains cannot distinguish between real and imagined events, we can harness this power for our benefit. By regularly practising visualization, we can create a mental environment that is conducive to calmness, confidence and healing.

For anyone looking to incorporate visualization into their daily life, the key is consistency. Just like any habit, the more you practise, the more natural it becomes. You can start with just a few minutes a day, using a guided recording or simply focusing on a mental image that brings you peace. Remember, it's not about forcing yourself to see something that isn't there; it's about allowing your mind to explore a new, more peaceful reality—one image at a time.

33

Positive Affirmation or Autosuggestions

Many times, our thoughts become our greatest source of stress. While the present situation may be starkly different, better and peaceful, it is our thoughts about the future or the past that create suffering.

Positive affirmations and autosuggestions are not just about saying nice words—they are about consciously and intentionally choosing thoughts that reshape our reality. This practice has roots in ancient wisdom, modern psychology and scientific research, showing us that our words and thoughts have the power to create our experiences and even change the state of our nervous system. But how does it work? And why do our thoughts and words matter so much?

Every thought we think, every word we speak, sends signals throughout our body. These signals influence our nervous system, triggering either a state of calm (PNS) or a state of stress (SNS).

When we repeat negative thoughts like, 'I'm not good enough,' 'I'll never get better' or 'I'm worthless,' our body perceives these thoughts as threats, triggering a stress response. This releases stress hormones, like cortisol, which keeps us in a heightened state of alertness and anxiety.

Conversely, when we use positive affirmations such as, 'I am safe,' 'I am healing' or 'I am worthy of love,' we can shift the nervous system from a fight-or-flight state into a state of rest-and-digest. This is the power of positive self-talk and autosuggestions—helping to bring the body back into a balanced, calmer state. It's like a reset button for the mind and body, allowing us to breathe deeper, think clearer and manage stress more effectively.

The Science Behind Positive Affirmations

When certain thoughts are repeated with intention, they can create new neural pathways in the brain. This process is known as neuroplasticity—the brain's ability to change and adapt, based on new thoughts and experiences.

Studies published on PubMed and by NCBI have shown that self-affirmations can activate brain regions associated with reward and positive self-views, helping individuals cope better with stress and improve emotional regulation (Cascio et al., 2016). These changes are not instant, but with repetition, the brain gradually adopts new, healthier thought patterns.

For example, if someone, who struggles with chronic pain, continually tells themselves, 'My body is healing, I am becoming stronger,' it can help their brain to focus on recovery rather than pain. This shift in focus can ease their perception of pain and reduce the stress response, allowing the body to focus more energy on healing. Research in the *Journal of Psychosomatic Research* has shown that positive affirmations can lead to improved health outcomes, even among those dealing with serious illnesses (Sherman et al., 2013).

Thoughts Create Feelings, Feelings Create Actions and Actions Create Experiences

Our thoughts shape our reality in a very direct way. Here's how the cycle works:

Thoughts create feelings → feelings lead to actions → actions generate results → results create our experiences.

When our thoughts are predominantly negative, they evoke feelings of fear, anxiety and sadness. These feelings influence our actions—perhaps causing us to isolate ourselves, avoid challenges or lash out at others. These actions then shape our results, often leading to experiences of loneliness, failure or strained relationships, which reinforce the negative thoughts that started the cycle.

However, by using positive affirmations, we can intervene in this cycle. For example, if someone continually thinks, 'I am useless and good for nothing,' they may begin to act in ways that align with this belief—avoiding opportunities, missing out on joy or settling for unhealthy relationships.

On the other hand, affirmations like, 'I am capable, I am enough,' can help them shift their mindset, thus enabling them to take small steps toward better actions and, eventually, more positive experiences. It's about using words to rewrite the script that plays in our minds.

Throughout history, various religious texts have emphasized the power of words. The Bible states, 'Death and life are in the power of the tongue' (Proverbs 18:21), suggesting that the words we speak can either uplift or bring us down. This ancient wisdom parallels modern psychology, which acknowledges the profound impact of self-talk on our mental and physical well-being. Words are not empty sounds; they carry energy and meaning. They have the power to either make or break us.

The phrase 'abracadabra', often associated with magic, has roots in Aramaic, meaning, 'I create as I speak.' It's a reminder that our words have creative power. Our tongue can become a wand, shaping our reality by influencing our thoughts and beliefs. When we speak kindly to ourselves, our mind begins to believe those words, creating a sense of inner peace even amidst external chaos.

Affirmations Are Not Mere Words: The Importance of Feeling and Belief

For affirmations to be truly effective, they must be spoken with conviction and emotion. It's not about mindlessly repeating phrases—it's about feeling the energy behind the words. Imagine a couple where one partner says, 'I love you' out of habit, while another couple shares those words with deep emotion and connection. The difference lies in the energy and intent behind the words and how deeply they resonate.

Similarly, when practising affirmations, we need to connect with the feelings and meanings behind them. Saying 'I am healthy,' while feeling disconnected from the statement may not yield results. But when we close our eyes, take a deep breath and imagine the feeling of health and vitality flowing through our body, the affirmation takes on new power. It becomes a tool that not only shifts our thoughts but also influences our emotions and actions.

Reframing Negative Narratives

Imagine a teenager who constantly tells themselves, 'I'll never fit in, no one likes me.' These thoughts lead to feelings of loneliness and anxiety, which then shape their actions—avoiding social interactions, withdrawing from friends or acting defensive in conversations. As a result, they feel more isolated, which reinforces their initial thoughts of being unlikable.

Now, imagine if they begin to replace those thoughts with affirmations like, 'I am worthy of friendship' or 'I bring value to those around me.' At first, these words might feel untrue, but with repetition, the brain starts to adopt them as new beliefs. The teenager might then start smiling more, reaching out to others and showing kindness, which leads to positive social experiences. Over time, their reality shifts, simply because they changed their thoughts.

Renowned affirmation expert Louise Hay has long advocated for the power of words in healing. In her teachings, she emphasizes that 'The thoughts we think and the words we speak create our experiences.'

Dr Joe Dispenza, a well-known neuroscientist, further explores this concept by highlighting that 'You are the placebo.' He suggests that the mind can significantly influence the body's physiology, and by changing thoughts, one can change their biology. Dispenza's work demonstrates how powerful autosuggestions can be in shifting the brain's chemistry, which, in turn, affects the body's ability to heal.

For those facing health issues, relationship struggles or life's uncertainties, here are some affirmations that can support a shift towards healing and inner peace:

'Every day and in every way, I am getting better and better.'

'The divine intelligence in my body is working for me to heal and protect me.'

'I deserve and am worthy of love, happiness and abundant health.'

'I am protected, safe and guided.'

'I trust the process of life and know that I am being taken care of.'

'I am resilient, and I overcome challenges with grace.'

These affirmations, when repeated consistently and with feeling, can become a powerful anchor reflecting hope, healing and resilience. Speak the health, love, success, relationships and life you want.

34

Smart Fasting

Fasting, when approached with mindfulness and respect for the body's natural rhythms, is a powerful practice that can bring balance across our physical, mental and spiritual states. Yet, the beauty of fasting is often obscured by trends, diets and rigid structures.

Smart fasting is not about squeezing ourselves into a 16:8 box or starving ourselves until we're lightheaded; it's about honouring our body's needs for nourishment and rest. It's about listening to our bodies, acknowledging their signals and aligning with nature's cycles—most naturally, the circadian rhythm fast.

Circadian Fasting: The Most Natural and No-Nonsense Way to Fast

Circadian rhythm fasting represents the most intuitive and natural way to fast. This approach aligns our eating patterns with the cycles of the sun. It means making sunset your last meal and allowing your body to rest from the evening until sunrise. This practice typically results in a 12-hour fast, from dinner to breakfast, without the strain or discomfort often associated with more rigid fasting schedules.

Eating closer to sunset allows the body to focus on vital processes of elimination, repair and rejuvenation. When we allow our digestive system to rest, we free up energy that would be typically diverted towards digestion, redirecting it instead to healing and elimination. This gentle pause in feeding mirrors how our ancestors lived for centuries—long before modern conveniences made eating at all hours possible.

What we now call intermittent fasting or time-restricted eating is far from a novel concept. This way of living was embedded naturally in human existence through evolution. There were periods of feasting and periods of fasting, and our bodies adapted to this rhythm. Our ancestors didn't have the luxury of food delivery apps or the convenience of a store around every corner. Food was seasonal and its availability varied, making fasting a natural part of life.

In today's times, however, instant gratification is everywhere. The snack industry perpetuates the idea that we need a 4 p.m. snack, while food delivery apps ensure that a meal is never more than a few taps away. The constant need to munch has taken us away from our intuitive selves and our ability to eat only when our body truly requires nourishment. We've become accustomed to eating out of habit or emotion rather than genuine hunger.

As a result, many of us have lost touch with the natural signals our body gives us—the rumble of an empty stomach, the lightness that comes from true rest from food. In short, the feeling of true hunger. Yet, those who have embraced fasting often describe a return to these natural states. They speak of feeling calmer, more peaceful and more focused, experiencing improved sleep and even heightened creativity.

Fasting As a Protector: Activating the Body's Mechanisms

While abundance is often celebrated as a marker of prosperity, endless access to food can overwhelm the body's systems. In contrast, fasting triggers protective mechanisms that enhance our overall health. It is as if our body shifts into a maintenance mode. Research has shown that fasting activates genes and proteins associated with longevity, repair and stress resistance.

One such process, autophagy, involves cleaning out damaged cells and components, effectively allowing our body to repair itself. This process not only promotes cellular health but also supports mental clarity, mood regulation and longevity.

Fasting is not about deprivation; it is a powerful form of self-preservation and resilience. However, it's important to understand the delicate balance involved in fasting. While it has significant benefits, starvation or extreme fasting can lead to stress for the body. This stress, often perceived as a threat, engages the SNS—the 'fight-or-flight' response—triggering feelings of anxiety and discomfort.

The Calm Within: Vagus Nerve Activation and Spiritual Clarity

Fasting has been described as a practice that not only rests the digestive system but also calms the mind. Many individuals report feeling a deeper sense of calm and clarity during fasting. This is partly due to the activation of the vagus nerve, which plays a critical role in the PNS—the 'rest-and-digest' state. When the vagus nerve is activated, it helps down-regulate the nervous system, easing stress and promoting tranquillity. This activation may explain why fasting has been integral to spiritual practices across cultures, as it creates a profound connection between the mind and body, often leading to heightened spiritual awareness.

Throughout history, various religions have encouraged fasting not as an act of suffering, but as a means to achieve mental clarity and a closer connection to a higher power. In these fasted states, individuals often find themselves more attuned to their thoughts, emotions and the deeper questions of life. Fasting creates a space where distractions fade away, allowing for introspection and spiritual growth.

Fasting As a Trend: A Lost Art

Unfortunately, the art of fasting has been overshadowed by fads and competitive challenges, and that is where trends, such as the popular 16:8, fall short. Fasting has turned it into a race—who can fast the longest or who can endure the hardest hunger pangs. The essence of fasting is lost when we measure it against others' routines instead of tuning into our body's needs. There is no one size that fits all. For some, fasting for 16 hours might feel rejuvenating, but for others, it leads to irritability, dizziness, weakness and cravings.

The question arises: why should we all conform to a single fasting schedule when each of us is so different?

Everybody is unique, with different metabolic rates, activity levels and even emotional responses to food. For some individuals, a 14:10 or a 12:12 fasting window works beautifully, while others may thrive on a longer 18:6 or even a 24-hour intermittent fast.

The most sustainable and beneficial approach to fasting is one that suits you and works for you. It is intuitive in nature, which means it involves tuning into hunger cues rather than adhering to a rigid timetable. It encourages eating when genuinely hungry and allows the digestive system to rest when not. Studies have shown that individuals, who adopt a more intuitive approach to fasting, experience reduced anxiety and a greater ability to stick with the practice over time.

Experts in the field of fasting, such as Dr Satchin Panda and Dr Jason Fung, emphasize the importance of tailoring fasting practices to individual needs. They argue that there is no 'perfect' fasting window; rather, it's about listening to our bodies and finding a routine that feels both challenging and nurturing.

Scientific Research on Fasting

Numerous scientific studies support the myriad benefits of fasting. A systematic review published in *Nutrition Reviews* found that intermittent fasting can lead to weight loss, improved metabolic health and enhanced cardiovascular health. Additionally, research from the *Journal of Translational Medicine* has shown that fasting can improve insulin sensitivity and reduce markers of inflammation in the body.

Moreover, studies on caloric restriction, such as those conducted by researchers at the National Institute on Aging, indicate that fasting can extend the lifespan and promote healthy ageing. These findings emphasize that fasting is not merely a trend, but a profound practice grounded in science.

The impact of fasting on mental health is also noteworthy. A study published in *Scientific Reports* revealed that individuals, who engage in intermittent fasting, reported lower levels of anxiety and depression. The authors of the study suggested that the hormonal and metabolic changes associated with fasting might play a role in these improvements.

Ultimately, smart fasting is about finding balance—honouring the states between eating and resting, nourishment and elimination. It's not about depriving ourselves or pushing beyond our limits. When done right, fasting helps us tap into a state of calm, clarity and healing that no superfood or supplement can replicate. It should always be a practice that enhances our well-being, not one that adds stress to our lives.

35

Thought Checks, Pauses to Challenge and Reframe Negative Thoughts

Thoughts are powerful. They act as seeds for the emotions we experience and the actions we take. To feel happiness, sadness, anger or peace, we must first have thoughts that trigger these emotions. Neuroscientific research supports this connection: thoughts stimulate brain regions responsible for emotional regulation, creating a domino effect that affects our mood, behaviour and even our health.

But what happens when these thoughts become overwhelmingly negative? Often, persistent, unchallenged negative thoughts can spiral, feeding feelings of fear, anger, guilt and anxiety. This cycle activates our SNS—the 'fight-or-flight' response—keeping us on edge and under stress. While our survival instincts are essential, living in a prolonged fight-or-flight state disrupts the body's natural balance, impacting both mental and physical well-being. To break free from this cycle, science suggests that reframing negative thoughts, at their source, can shift our nervous system toward the 'rest-and-digest' mode, mediated by the PNS.

The Science Behind Reframing Thoughts

Psychologically, negative thoughts activate areas in the brain associated with threat detection and stress response, including the amygdala and hypothalamus. These brain regions prompt the release of cortisol and adrenaline, the body's primary stress hormones. Chronic activation of these pathways is linked to numerous adverse health outcomes, from cardiovascular disease to weakened immune function and cognitive decline.

When we intentionally pause and reframe our thoughts, however, we engage the brain's prefrontal cortex, the centre of rational thought, problem-solving and self-regulation.

Studies published on platforms like PubMed and by NCBI show that this intentional mental shift can lower stress levels by decreasing amygdala activation and strengthening prefrontal cortex engagement. As a result, this simple cognitive adjustment promotes a physiological shift toward the parasympathetic state, where the body can relax, digest and repair.

According to Dr Elizabeth Blackburn, a Nobel laureate in physiology and a prominent researcher on stress and cellular ageing, 'Every thought can contribute to our state of being, for better or worse.' Blackburn's research on telomeres—the protective caps on chromosomes that shorten with stress—demonstrates that chronic negative thinking can accelerate ageing at the cellular level, while a more balanced, reframed approach can preserve cellular health.

Why Thought Checks Matter: Our Brain's Reality Illusion

Experts, like Dr Joe Dispenza and Dr Daniel Goleman, emphasize that the mind often fails to differentiate between real and imagined stressors. When we visualize a worrisome situation, our bodies react as if it's genuinely happening, producing stress hormones and eliciting physical responses. This phenomenon is known as 'perceived threat' stress, where imagined dangers cause the same physiological reactions as actual threats.

This concept of 'perceived threat' stress helps explain why it's easy to get stuck in a loop of anxiety, fear or anger. When we constantly think, 'What if I fail at this?' or 'I'm not good enough,' our bodies interpret these statements as real, releasing stress hormones in response. Over time, this persistent stress keeps the body locked in the sympathetic state, unable to relax fully.

Research suggests that techniques like cognitive restructuring (reframing negative thoughts) can effectively reduce symptoms of anxiety and depression. For instance, a study published in *Cognitive Therapy and Research* found that participants, trained in reframing negative thoughts, showed a significant reduction in stress levels and improved overall well-being.

Another study conducted by the American Psychological Association (APA) concluded that individuals who regularly practise thought reframing, experience enhanced emotional resilience and are better equipped to handle life's challenges.

The evidence is compelling: challenging and reframing negative thoughts isn't just a mental exercise—it's a neurological intervention that can shift our body's stress response, protect cellular health and improve mental clarity and emotional stability.

Incorporating thought checks and reframing into daily life doesn't require significant time or resources. By making a habit of challenging and reframing our thoughts, we can gradually alter our mental patterns and promote a shift in our nervous system. Here's a practical approach:

1. **Pause and acknowledge:** When a negative thought surfaces, resist the urge to react immediately. Instead, pause and acknowledge it. Recognize it as just a thought—one version of reality, not an absolute truth.
2. **Challenge the thought:** Ask yourself if the thought is based on facts or assumptions. Negative thoughts are often exaggerated and may not reflect the real situation. Look for evidence to counter the negative thought.
3. **Reframe the thought:** Once you've challenged the negative thought, reframe it with a positive or neutral alternative. Shift from what you fear to what you want, and emphasize positive intentions.

4. **Practise regularly:** Consistency is crucial. Like any skill, the more frequently you practise thought checks and reframing, the more natural it will become, gradually rewiring your brain's response to stress.

Examples of Reframing Negative Thoughts

Here are some real-life scenarios and examples of reframing negative thoughts that can help regulate our nervous system:

- **Situation:** You're facing a health challenge and think, 'This is the end; my life will never be the same.'
- **Reframe:** 'This is difficult, but I can adapt. I will take the necessary steps to improve my health.'

- **Situation:** You experience a setback at work and think, 'I'm a failure; I'll never succeed.'
- **Reframe:** 'Everyone experiences setbacks. This is an opportunity to learn and grow. I'll apply what I've learned and keep moving forward.'

- **Situation:** You feel overwhelmed by family responsibilities and think, 'I can't handle this; it's too much.'
- **Reframe:** 'I've managed challenges before. I can break things down, prioritize and take it one step at a time.'

Each reframed thought acknowledges the situation, without spiralling into fear or anxiety, thereby creating a sense of control and inner peace. By practising this technique regularly, we can condition our brains to respond with calmness and resilience rather than stress and reactivity.

As we make thought reframing a habit, we gradually increase our brain's ability to shift into a parasympathetic state, promoting relaxation and physiological repair. Over time, this practice can decrease blood pressure, lower heart rate, improve digestion, enhance immunity and reduce overall inflammation. Research shows that regular engagement in cognitive reframing can improve sleep quality, reduce symptoms of chronic pain and lower the risks associated with stress-induced diseases.

Psychologist Dr Richard Davidson, a pioneer in the study of emotions and the brain, emphasizes, 'Our emotional style is not set in stone; we can change it.' His work highlights that even people with a tendency towards negative thoughts can reshape their mental and emotional patterns with consistent practice, leading to a greater sense of calm and resilience.

36

Using Food as Medicine

The connection between nutrition and emotional well-being is deeper than many realize. Nature, in its infinite wisdom, has provided us with foods rich in nutrients that can help us achieve a state of calm. By supplying essential raw materials, certain foods support the production of neurotransmitters—molecules that communicate between neurons and play a critical role in regulating mood and the state of our nervous system.

Certain foods contain nutrients that directly influence neurotransmitter synthesis, such as serotonin, dopamine, oxytocin, endorphins, GABA and acetylcholine. Neurotransmitters are chemical messengers that facilitate communication within the brain and between the brain and the body. How we feel, think and react are largely determined by the interplay of neurotransmitters. Understanding how our food choices affect these messengers can empower us to make decisions that enhance our mental and emotional health.

- **Serotonin:** Often called the 'feel-good' neurotransmitter, serotonin is crucial for mood stabilization, well-being and happiness. Approximately 90 per cent of serotonin is produced in the gut, highlighting the importance of gut health in mood regulation. Tryptophan, an amino acid, found in foods like turkey, eggs, salmon and nuts, is a precursor to serotonin. Probiotics in yoghurt and fermented foods, like kimchi and sauerkraut, also support serotonin production by maintaining a healthy gut microbiome.

- **Dopamine:** This neurotransmitter is linked to reward, pleasure and motivation. Foods rich in tyrosine, such as almonds, avocados, bananas and dark chocolate or cacao, are essential for dopamine synthesis. Research suggests that a diet rich in quality protein can enhance dopamine production. Omega-3 fatty acids, found in fatty fish like salmon and mackerel, also help maintain the integrity of dopamine receptors.
- **Oxytocin:** Known as the 'love hormone', oxytocin builds feelings of connection and trust. While it is often released during social bonding, certain foods can promote its secretion indirectly by supporting a calm and balanced mood. Magnesium-rich foods like leafy greens, nuts and seeds help reduce stress, creating conditions conducive to oxytocin release.
- **Endorphins:** These natural painkillers are released in response to pain and stress, creating a sense of euphoria. Foods like dark chocolate and spicy foods containing capsaicin, such as green chilies and cayenne pepper, can stimulate endorphin release. Studies indicate that combining moderate exercise with these foods can significantly boost endorphin production.
- **GABA:** GABA is an inhibitory neurotransmitter that calms the mind. Foods like green tea (rich in L-theanine), fermented foods, like kimchi, sauerkraut and kefir, and certain nuts can naturally increase GABA levels. L-theanine in green tea enhances alpha brainwave activity, promoting a relaxed, yet alert, state. Research suggests that regular consumption of L-theanine can improve focus and reduce anxiety.
- **Acetylcholine:** This neurotransmitter supports learning, memory and attention. Choline, a precursor to acetylcholine, is abundant in foods like eggs, liver

and soybeans. Adequate choline intake is essential for maintaining cognitive function and focus.

Additional Nutrients to Note:

- **Apigenin:** A flavonoid found in chamomile, parsley and celery, apigenin is known for its anxiolytic (anxiety-reducing) properties. Chamomile tea, rich in apigenin, has been used, for centuries, as a natural remedy for anxiety and insomnia.
- **Probiotics and Prebiotics:** A healthy gut microbiome is key to mental health, as the gut–brain axis significantly influences mood regulation. Probiotics (live beneficial bacteria found in fermented foods) and prebiotics (fibres that nourish these bacteria) can enhance gut health and promote neurotransmitter production, like serotonin.

Now, imagine a diet deprived of these nutrients—the very building blocks of vital neurotransmitters. This is the consequence of consuming junk, packaged, processed and ultra-processed foods. It's no surprise, then, why a nutrient-dense diet is essential not just for physical health but for emotional well-being, too.

I had the privilege of hosting Dr Uma Naidoo, a Harvard-trained psychiatrist, nutrition specialist and author of *This Is Your Brain on Food*, on my podcast. During our conversation, she shared her insights into the connection between food and emotions. She explained how certain foods can act as natural antidepressants by nourishing the gut microbiome and boosting neurotransmitter production. Hosting her on my podcast served as a powerful reminder that food is a controllable factor in our lives—one that can significantly influence how we feel each day.

In our practice of Integrative and Lifestyle Medicine, it's critical to focus on cellular nutrition—ensuring that the body receives the nutrients it needs to function optimally at a molecular level. Sometimes, mood imbalances stem from genuine nutrient deficiencies. For example, a lack of magnesium can impair serotonin production, leading to symptoms of anxiety and irritability. Similarly, deficiencies in B vitamins, particularly B6 and B12, can disrupt the synthesis of neurotransmitters like dopamine and serotonin.

This is not to undermine the importance of medication when needed, but to emphasize that nutrition forms the foundation of our health. Addressing the basics is essential.

Food is one of the most controllable aspects of our lives and our emotional health. Let's use this power wisely.

37

Limiting Junk, Packaged, Processed and Ultra-Processed Foods

Is there even one scientific article or paper showing that junk food is beneficial for health? No. So, it's simple. While people often demand research to validate what's healthy or not, sometimes we just need to use a bit of common sense—actually, loads of it. We all know that consistently consuming junk, processed and ultra-processed foods does more harm than good. This isn't just about chips and packaged snacks, but also includes overly processed vegan and vegetarian options like mock meats, processed meats and cold cuts. Keep it real—whatever you choose to eat should nourish your body.

Junk Food: A Modern-Day Stressor on the Body

Junk food, fast food and ultra-processed foods are not truly 'food'—they're chemical concoctions designed for profit, not health. These foods are filled with sugar, unhealthy fats, artificial additives and preservatives that stress our bodies in ways we often underestimate. When consumed regularly, they create a cascade of negative effects, including inflammation, free radical production, hyperactivity and relentless cravings.

What Makes Junk Food Addictive?

Ever wondered why it's so hard to stop at just a handful of chips or a cookie? Junk food is designed to be addictive, with carefully balanced amounts of salt, sugar and fat. These three ingredients are 'tastemakers', hitting the sweet spot of flavour that keeps you coming back for more. The food industry employs this addictive trifecta to keep you hooked, and it's not an accident—it's science. Studies have shown that combining sugar, fat and salt stimulates the brain's reward centre, just like addictive substances do.

The fats used in these foods are often the lowest quality, highly refined and processed. The sugars are a mix of different forms, including high-fructose corn syrup, which is much sweeter than regular sugar and more harmful. Hidden sugars and large quantities of salt complete this cocktail, tricking your taste buds and keeping you reaching for more. But it doesn't end there.

When you consume sugary or refined foods, your blood sugar spikes rapidly. This gives you a quick burst of energy, but that high is fleeting. Soon, blood sugar levels plummet, leading to the notorious 'sugar crash'. This crash makes you feel irritable, tired and even hungrier than before. This is why an hour after eating a sugar-laden snack, you might find yourself reaching for yet another. The brain craves sugar because it releases dopamine—a neurotransmitter associated with pleasure. This is why sugar can be so addictive.

A study published in the *American Journal of Clinical Nutrition* found that high glycaemic index foods, like sugar and refined grains, activate areas of the brain linked to reward and craving, much like addictive drugs. But this is not a harmless craving. The constant cycle of sugar highs and lows can lead to insulin resistance, increased body fat and even cognitive decline, over time.

Inflammation, Free Radicals and Their Impact on Health

Junk food doesn't just wreak havoc on your waistline—it creates inflammation throughout the body. Processed foods are often loaded with refined carbohydrates, trans-fats and artificial additives that contribute to oxidative stress and inflammation. This chronic inflammation is a known contributor to conditions like obesity, diabetes, heart disease and mental health issues, such as anxiety and depression.

Inflammation triggers the release of cytokines—proteins that can affect brain function. When inflammation levels are high, it becomes harder for the body to regulate stress, leading to a hyperactive nervous system. This means that while you're indulging in these comfort foods, you're actually putting your body in a state of heightened stress, counteracting the very comfort you're seeking.

Urban Malnutrition: A Hidden Crisis

Today, malnutrition is not just a rural issue anymore. Even people living in cities, with access to a variety of foods, can suffer from malnutrition. This might sound counterintuitive, but it is a reality. Urban malnutrition stems from consuming calorie-dense but nutrient-poor diets, like those high in fast food and processed snacks. These foods often lack essential vitamins and minerals, leading to 'hidden hunger'.

You can have a full stomach and still be malnourished if the food you're eating lacks the nutrients needed for optimal health. This manifests as fatigue, poor concentration, weakened immunity and emotional instability. A study by the World Health Organization (WHO) highlighted that urban populations are increasingly facing the double burden of malnutrition—where undernutrition coexists with obesity and metabolic disorders.

Dr Mark Hyman, a pioneer in functional medicine, often discusses how modern processed diets contribute to inflammation and emotional instability. He emphasizes that the highly processed nature of today's food is not compatible with our body's needs for stability and balance. According to him, the key is to eat whole, minimally processed foods that support our gut health and, in turn, our mental clarity and mood stability. A study published in *Nature Reviews*

Neuroscience supports this, showing that a healthy gut microbiome is crucial for maintaining a balanced mood and reducing anxiety.

So, what happens when you finally say goodbye to these addictive foods? The results can be magical. From increased energy levels to improved mood and a boost in immunity, the benefits are profound. The body has an incredible ability to heal when given the right fuel.

For many years, we have been doing various global challenges on social media for cutting processed foods just for three days. People who have participated in these global, sugar-free challenges report feeling lighter, more energetic and mentally clear within just a few days of cutting out processed foods.

One participant shared, 'All I did was cut out sugar and add some moderate exercise. Within a couple of weeks, I felt lighter, my brain fog was gone and the puffiness in my body and face had reduced.' These real-life experiences highlight the immense power of reducing or eliminating junk and processed foods from our diets.

Why do so many people continue to consume junk food, despite its known risks? The answer lies in aggressive marketing, deceptive labels and misleading information. Slick advertisements and endorsements by role models make these foods appear as harmless treats. Yet, the reality is far different. Behind the colourful packaging lies a cocktail of chemicals, unhealthy fats, sugars and artificial colours.

The truth is, junk food, fast food and ultra-processed foods are not real food—they are engineered to be addictive, cheap and profitable. There is no middle ground. Even claims like 'baked, not fried', '20% less fat' or 'fruit-flavoured' don't change the fact that these products still contribute to inflammation and poor health.

So, what should be your next step? The first and most powerful step you can take is to clean out your kitchen—get rid of the junk in your fridge, pantry and snack drawer. It may feel difficult initially, but out of sight is out of mind.

Removing these temptations makes it easier to make better choices and creates space for nourishing, whole foods that support your well-being.

It's time to reject smart marketing and embrace smart eating, using a whole load of common sense.

38

Deep and Slow Breathing

Breathing is the first thing that goes out of balance when we experience stress. For example, consider how an oxygen mask is the first thing administered to an accident victim when they are rushed into the hospital. While this is in response to physical trauma more than emotional stress, the body's reaction to different kinds of stress—be it physical, emotional or psychological—is remarkably similar. The first step is always to stabilize breathing, because when a body experiences trauma, breathing is often the first function that becomes erratic. By providing an oxygen mask, medical professionals aim to bring the breath back to balance, creating a foundation for further care.

Whether it's a moment of intense pressure, a stressful event or a sudden shock, our breathing patterns shift instantly—often becoming shallow, rapid or even erratic. This change is an automatic response to stress, signalling the body to prepare for action. However, just as breathing is the first thing to change when we experience stress, it is also the first thing that can bring us back to a balanced state, or homoeostasis, when we focus on it.

Breathing is not just about taking in oxygen; it directly affects the balance of the ANS, which comprises the SNS (fight-or-flight) and PNS (rest-and-digest) branches. Deep, slow breaths activate the PNS, signalling to the body that it is safe, which, in turn, reduces cortisol and adrenaline levels.

A study published in *Frontiers in Human Neuroscience* explored how slow-paced breathing activates the PNS, enhancing feelings of relaxation and calmness. When we engage in deep, conscious breathing, we activate the PNS, which signals to the body that it is safe. This allows the body to move from a state of heightened alertness to a state of relaxation and recovery. It's akin to hitting the 'reset' button, allowing us to regain control over our physiological state.

A powerful technique within deep breathing is the practice of slowing down the breath—extending the duration of inhales and, even more importantly, the exhales. The ancient yoga texts suggest a breathing ratio of 1:2, meaning that the length of the exhale should be twice that of the inhale. This method of slowing down the exhale induces a state of relaxation, as it directly stimulates the vagus nerve, a key player in the PNS.

This is beautifully encapsulated in the teachings of Patanjali. The *Yoga Sutras* emphasize the importance of breath in calming the mind:

Patanjali Yoga Sutra 1.34:
प्रच्छर्दनविधारणाभ्यां वा प्राणस्य।

Transliteration:
Pracchardana-Vidharanabhyam Va Pranasya.

Translation:
By exhalation and retention of breath, the mind can be calmed.

From a scientific perspective, longer exhales help to reduce the heart rate, enhance heart rate variability and decrease cortisol levels in the bloodstream. A study in the *Journal of Alternative and Complementary Medicine* found that when participants practised slow exhalation breathing techniques, their heart rate decreased, and their sense of calmness increased. Slow exhales help to tap into the body's natural relaxation response.

How Deep Breathing Works: The Science Behind the Calm

When we take in a deep breath, our diaphragm—our primary breathing muscle—contracts, creating more space in the chest cavity and allowing the lungs to expand fully. This process increases oxygen levels in the blood and reduces carbon dioxide. As the levels of carbon dioxide drop, so do cortisol and adrenaline levels, telling the body that it is safe. This does not mean that the stressor has disappeared, but rather that our body's physiological response is better equipped to handle it. In essence, we become more resilient in the face of challenges, entering a state where we can 'rest-and-digest' rather than 'fight or flee'.

A study in the *Frontiers in Psychology* found that participants who practised deep breathing for over eight weeks experienced significant reductions in cortisol levels and perceived stress. This demonstrates that regular deep breathing can support long-term stress management and resilience.

While deep breathing doesn't eliminate the external stressors in our lives, it enhances our ability to cope with them. It allows our body to handle stress better by creating a physiological environment that is conducive to relaxation. In other words, deep breathing makes us more resilient to life's challenges, enabling us to face stressors with greater calm and clarity.

The Role of Pranayama and Yogic Breathing Techniques

Pranayama, the ancient practice of breath control in yoga, is a beautiful and powerful tool to help bring about balance and homoeostasis in the body. These breathing exercises help regulate the flow of energy, or *prana*, and have a direct impact on our nervous system.

Research published in the *International Journal of Yoga* emphasizes that pranayama practices can improve HRV, a key indicator of stress resilience and autonomic balance.

Here are some of the most effective pranayama techniques for down-regulating an overactive nervous system:

1. **Box Breathing**: This technique involves inhaling for a count of four, holding the breath for four, exhaling for four and holding the exhale for another four counts. This simple, yet powerful, method helps to slow down the breath, bringing the heart rate down and calming the mind.
2. **4–7–8 Breathing**: This exercise involves inhaling for 4 seconds, holding the breath for 7 seconds and exhaling slowly for 8 seconds. It is known for its ability to quickly activate the PNS, helping to bring about a sense of deep relaxation.
3. ***Anulom Vilom* (Alternate Nostril Breathing)**: In this practice, you alternate the breath between the left and right nostrils, which helps to balance the left and right hemispheres of the brain. It is particularly effective for managing anxiety and creating a sense of inner balance.
4. **Diaphragmatic Breathing**: Also known as belly breathing, this involves breathing deeply into the abdomen, allowing the diaphragm to engage fully. It encourages a full oxygen exchange, slows the heart rate and stabilizes blood pressure.

Numerous scientific studies have explored the benefits of deep breathing and pranayama for stress management. Research published by NCBI and PubMed highlights how conscious breathing can positively influence HRV. Higher HRV is associated with a more relaxed state, and deep breathing exercises have been shown to improve HRV, thereby enhancing resilience to stress.

Experts in the field of breathing, like Dr Richard Brown and Dr Patricia Gerbarg, emphasize the importance of breath work in managing anxiety and trauma. Their research has shown that breathing exercises can enhance vagal tone, which is critical for regulating the PNS. By increasing vagal tone, we can transition from a state of stress to one of relaxation more easily.

Breathing is a vital tool that we can harness daily to maintain a balanced nervous system. Whether we are eating, sleeping or facing a challenging situation, being mindful of our breath can help us stay in the right physiological state.

For instance, before meals, taking a few deep breaths can shift us into the parasympathetic state, allowing us to engage fully in the 'rest-and-digest' mode. This helps our body break down, digest and assimilate nutrients effectively, preventing issues like bloating, indigestion and acid reflux.

Deep breathing, before and after meals, serves as a small, but powerful, habit that can transform the way we digest food and experience mealtime. It's a reminder that 'vitamin O'—oxygen—is essential, and slow, deep breaths can prepare our bodies to rest-and-digest with ease.

That said, just as any other skill, mastering the art of deep breathing takes practice and consistency. Make small wins, like taking a moment to breathe deeply before a meal or during a stressful moment. This can accumulate over time, leading to profound shifts in our well-being.

While stress will always be a part of life, the power of our breath allows us to face it from a place of balance and strength. So, take a deep breath, and remember: your breath is your ally in the journey towards balance and well-being.

39

Spending Time in Nature

Nature has an incredible ability to shift us from a state of stress to one of relaxation. No matter how much stress fills your life, spending time in nature can bring you back to a place of balance and calm. On my trip to Finland, surrounded by endless forests and serene lakes, I could feel the shift from stress to tranquillity almost instantly.

While nature may not solve your problems, it does change what happens inside your body, helping you return to homoeostasis—the state where all the magic of healing happens. In this state, your body works in harmony; but when you're out of balance, your body can become its own gangster, yielding the weapon of uncontrolled inflammation and paving the way for numerous lifestyle issues.

Wherever you are in the world, and no matter how busy your day is, make it a priority to spend time in nature. Some may say, 'I live in a city; I don't have access to nature.' But nature is everywhere—you just have to find it. It could be as simple as sunlight streaming into your home, sitting by a window and feeling the fresh air, or watching the sunrise without the distraction of your phone. Even having plants or flowers around your house brings nature closer to you.

If you can, take walks in parks, spend time near trees or engage in grounding activities on grass or at the beach. If you're lucky enough to live in a place surrounded by nature, make the most of it. Don't let yourself be stuck indoors, glued to your phone or tablet, missing out on the free and powerful gifts that nature offers—gifts more healing than any drug.

You might notice that in a city, people often seem more aggressive or easily stressed. That's because they are constantly in a fight-or-flight mode, craving stimulants like coffee or the dopamine hits from social gatherings. But when you're in nature, everything changes. Your mood, behaviour, energy and even your thoughts become more peaceful because nature profoundly affects every cell in your body. In the city, I notice how much more on the go or on edge I can become, as opposed to when I am in nature, and everything changes.

When in nature, you may find that you no longer need external stimulants because your body naturally balances itself. Serotonin, dopamine and other feel-good chemicals are all positively influenced by nature.

So, what are your plans to connect with nature? Even if you live in a bustling city, make time for weekend getaways to places where you can immerse yourself in nature. Plan your holidays around natural settings that allow you to recharge and return feeling renewed. The human body, mind and soul thrive in nature, so make sure you create that opportunity for yourself.

Early Humans: Their Connection to Nature

Early humans had a deep, reverent connection to the natural world around them, often worshiping natural elements and forces as sacred beings. They saw themselves as part of a larger ecosystem rather than separate from it, recognizing that their survival depended on nature's rhythms and resources. Rivers, mountains, trees and celestial bodies, like the sun and moon, were all seen as divine manifestations, and rituals were performed to honour these natural entities. This worship wasn't only about fear or gratitude; it was about seeing the interconnectedness of all life.

In ancient Indian philosophy, this connection evolved into a sophisticated understanding known as the concept of the *Panchamahabhuta*, or the Five Great Elements. These are believed to be the fundamental building blocks of all creation, from the human body to the cosmos.

The Five Elements in Nature and the Human Body

***Prithvi* (Earth)**

The earth element represents solidity, stability and support. Ancient people relied on the earth for food, shelter and sustenance. In the human body, prithvi corresponds to all solid structures: bones, teeth, muscles and tissues. Worshipping the earth as a mother goddess, early societies developed an understanding of farming, soil fertility and cycles of growth.

***Apas* (Water)**

Water was revered as a life-giving force, symbolizing flow, adaptability and purification. In human anatomy, apas governs bodily fluids like blood, lymph and digestive juices. Ancient civilizations worshipped rivers as deities, understanding that clean water was essential for health and survival. Many cultures performed water rituals to invoke blessings, purify the soul and maintain harmony with this element.

***Agni* (Fire)**

Fire represents transformation, energy and illumination. It holds a special place as both a creator and destroyer, offering warmth, protection and the ability to cook food. Fire's connection to the sun, lightning and controlled flames was sacred, with agni seen as a bridge between humans and the divine in Vedic traditions. The human body uses fire in the form of metabolism—the digestive fire *(jatharagni)* that transforms food into energy.

***Vayu* (Air)**

Air represents movement, breath and life force. For early people, air was seen as both a vital need and an invisible force carrying messages. In humans, vayu is the breath, essential for life, and the energy behind movement and circulation.

Many ancient cultures practised breath-focused rituals and meditations, understanding that breathing was a bridge between the body and spirit.

Akasha **(Ether/Space)**
Space is the subtlest element, representing the potential for everything to exist. Akasha is what holds everything together, encompassing all other elements within it. In the human body, Akasha is the space within—our sense of hearing, consciousness and inner potential. Ether allows communication and awareness, grounding the mind's subtle qualities and giving room for thoughts and feelings to exist.

Worship and Reverence for the Elements

Early rituals often involved offering elements back to themselves: fire rituals *(yagna)* as offerings to agni, water ceremonies for rivers and burying seeds and gifts into the earth. These acts were based on the understanding that everything is interconnected and harmony could be achieved only when humans respected and honoured the balance of nature. These traditions of worship can be seen in Hindu, Greek, Native American, African and many indigenous cultures worldwide, each with unique interpretations of the elements but with the shared respect for nature as sacred.

The Panchamahabhuta philosophy also extends to Ayurveda, where each element corresponds to the body's different energies or 'doshas' *(Vata, Pitta* and *Kapha)*. Ayurveda teaches that health is achieved by maintaining a balance of the five elements, understanding how they affect our bodies, minds and environments.

For instance:

- Earth (Kapha) provides structure and stability.
- Water (Kapha and Pitta) offers nourishment and flow.
- Fire (Pitta) transforms and digests.

- Air (Vata) facilitates movement and flexibility.
- Space (Vata) enables awareness and consciousness.

Try to be as one as you can with nature in your daily life; the benefits will last for a lifetime.

40

The Joy of Anticipation

Anticipation has a unique power that drives us as human beings, offering a sense of hope and excitement even amidst the most challenging times. Be it a vacation, a gathering with loved ones or a simple weekend break—the joy of looking forward to something acts as a gentle, yet powerful, tonic that helps us manage stress, balance our nervous system and transition from an upregulated, dysregulated state to a more harmonious one.

But how does this process work? What happens within our brain and body when we have something to look forward to? And how can it be used as a tool in therapeutic practices, even for those facing severe challenges, like cancer?

Anticipation and the Human Brain: The Neuroscience of Looking Forward

Anticipation is more than just a mental state; it's a biological process that deeply influences our brain and body. When we look forward to something positive, our brain releases dopamine—a neurotransmitter associated with pleasure, motivation and reward. Dopamine is produced in regions like the ventral tegmental area (VTA) and is released into the nucleus accumbens, a core part of the brain's reward system. This process creates a sense of eagerness and excitement, energizing us to pursue our goals and dreams.

Anticipation can also trigger the release of endorphins—natural painkillers in the body—that not only improve our mood, but also help us manage stress more effectively. This anticipation-induced chemical boost helps shift us from a heightened SNS state, where stress dominates, to a more relaxed PNS state, creating a sense of calmness and balance. Our body perceives a positive future outcome, and this state of calmness slows our heart rate, promotes deeper breathing and reduces cortisol levels.

In our practice too, we encourage our patients to talk about their dreams, goals or travel plans. It is a powerful way to shift their focus away from pain and uncertainty. When we ask a cancer patient, 'What would you like to do once you're in remission?' or 'Where would you love to travel when you feel better?' we invite their minds to visualize a future beyond their current struggle.

This forward-looking mindset can create a powerful shift in the brain's chemistry. By focusing on the anticipation of better days, the patient's brain releases dopamine, which not only elevates their mood, but also provides a sense of motivation and resilience.

For example, a patient undergoing chemotherapy may find comfort in thinking about a beach trip they plan to take once their treatment concludes. The very act of imagining the warm sand, the sound of the waves and the feeling of the sun on their skin can lift their spirits and provide a temporary escape from their current reality. This simple shift in focus can reduce their perception of pain, alleviate anxiety and help them cope better with the physical and emotional strain of treatment.

It's not only grand plans that bring joy; even small, regular plans can create a sense of anticipation that uplifts us. Think of the excitement of planning a weekend hike, a dinner with friends or even the simple joy of ordering a new book and eagerly awaiting its arrival. These small moments of looking forward to something also create pockets of relief from stress.

A study published in the *Journal of Positive Psychology* highlighted that people derive greater satisfaction from **anticipating a future experience than from anticipating a material purchase.** This suggests that experiences—like a planned day out or a creative project—carry more emotional weight in our brains than objects. This anticipation triggers a process called 'prospection', where we mentally time travel to future moments, which can provide solace during periods of stress.

Several studies have explored the benefits of anticipation on stress management and emotional well-being:

- A study published in *Frontiers in Human Neuroscience* found that anticipation of positive events can significantly reduce the stress response by increasing levels of serotonin, another neurotransmitter known for its role in mood regulation. Serotonin helps balance the nervous system, promoting a calm and steady mood.
- Research on *Applied Research in Quality of Life* has shown that looking forward to a vacation can improve the mood and reduce stress for weeks before the trip itself, indicating that the mere act of planning and anticipating positive experiences has a tangible impact on our well-being.
- A study in *Frontiers in Behavioral Neuroscience* emphasized the role of the prefrontal cortex in creating positive anticipation. It explained how the prefrontal cortex works in tandem with the amygdala, a part of the brain involved in processing fear and anxiety, to create a sense of hope and balance, even in the face of challenges.

Here are some ways to keep the mind focused on the positives ahead:

1. **Plan a weekly ritual:** Whether it's a Sunday morning walk, a Friday movie night or a special meal, having

something to look forward to each week can create a sense of rhythm and balance.

2. **Visualize future joys:** Spend a few minutes each day visualizing a positive event you are looking forward to. Imagine the details vividly—the sights, sounds and feelings—allowing your brain to tap into the reward system.
3. **Keep a 'Looking Forward' journal:** Write down one thing each day that you are excited about, no matter how small. This practice can shift your focus away from stressors and bring a sense of gratitude and anticipation.

By tapping into our innate ability to look forward to better days, we can navigate life's challenges with greater ease and grace. For those going through hardships, like a serious illness or daily stresses, anticipation becomes a light at the end of the tunnel—a reminder that there is a future beyond the present moment.

41

Slowing Down

In a world that glorifies speed, where hustle is often mistaken for progress, there lies a hidden truth: real magic happens when we slow down. Slowing down isn't about giving up our dreams or ambitions; it's about savouring the journey, reconnecting with our inner selves and allowing life to unfold with intention.

When we are constantly rushing, juggling tasks and feeling the pressure to keep up, our sympathetic nervous system remains overactive, flooding our bodies with stress hormones like adrenaline and cortisol. This state is vital in emergencies, but chronic activation wears us down, leading to anxiety, burnout and even physical illnesses.

On the other hand, slowing down allows us to tap into the parasympathetic state. This is where the body begins to repair, digest and heal. In this state, our breathing slows, our heart rate steadies and blood flow is directed to our organs and digestive system. It's a state that promotes longevity, helps in rejuvenating cells and bringing mental clarity.

Centenarians—those who live beyond 100 years—have long intrigued scientists. Many studies have explored the habits of these long-lived individuals, revealing a fascinating trend: they live in a state of unhurried ease. Studies published in the *Frontiers in Endocrinology* have shown that people who live longer tend to have lower levels of chronic stress and place a high value on relationships, time in nature and unhurried activities. In a study conducted in the Okinawa region of Japan, known for its population of long-lived individuals, researchers found that slowing down daily routines, such as taking time for meals and practising mindful movement like Tai Chi, contributes to both longevity and health. These practices promote a parasympathetic state, reducing oxidative stress and inflammation, which are key factors in ageing. Additionally, research from the American Heart Association has demonstrated that slowing down through practices like mindful breathing and meditation can significantly lower blood pressure and improve HRV—markers that indicate better ANS regulation.

Slowing down is not merely a personal preference but a science-backed approach to better health. Constantly rushing and multitasking can lead to what scientists refer to as 'allostatic load', which is essentially the wear and tear on the body due to chronic stress exposure. This can accelerate ageing by shortening telomeres, the protective caps on our chromosomes. Studies published in *Neuroscience & Biobehavioral Reviews* have found that a high allostatic load is linked with accelerated ageing, cognitive decline and increased risks of chronic diseases. In contrast, slowing down helps reduce this physiological burden. When we take time to rest, the body can repair damaged cells, balance hormones and restore homoeostasis. It's like giving the car a chance to cool down instead of constantly revving the engine. This reduction in stress hormones not only improves mood and mental clarity but also has a profound impact on longevity.

I call this way of living SlowFlow. It's a mindset and a lifestyle that allows us to be ambitious and dream big, but to pursue those dreams in a state of flow rather than frenzy. In the SlowFlow state of mind, we start to allow our thoughts, our energy and our authentic selves to flow. Blood flows more freely, stress melts away and everything aligns into a state of natural harmony.

When we slow down, we become more attuned to the subtle lessons life offers. We learn to appreciate the beauty in small moments, like the warmth of the sun on our face, or the intricate patterns of raindrops on a window. Slowing down doesn't mean that we stop aspiring; it means that we enjoy the process of growth, embrace the lessons from our mistakes and transform our flaws into strengths. It's about achieving without losing our health, our peace or our relationships.

My Journey with SlowFlow: Learning to Pause

I have always taken pride in the way I live my life. With over a thousand patients in my programmes and daily consultations with clients worldwide, many might think that I should feel rushed, wishing for more hours in my day. But I've found that 24 hours is just right—when used thoughtfully. Nature follows a 24-hour circadian rhythm, aligning with the rise and fall of the sun, and I strive to live in sync with this natural flow.

My time on social media is calculated. I use it to post, educate and learn, but then I log off. It's not a space where I seek validation or compare myself with others. I set clear intentions each day for what I want to share and learn, and I stick to that. Mindless scrolling has never been my thing; it adds no value to my well-being.

But it wasn't until a cyclone struck Goa, cutting off electricity and Wi-Fi for six days, that I truly realized the power of disconnecting. Those days were like a retreat, with no screens to distract me, only the simplicity of life: family time, the joy of reading books and the raw beauty of nature outside my window. It felt like a return to normal—a normal where thoughts are clear, energy flows effortlessly and the mind feels truly rested. I slept deeply, woke up naturally with the sunrise and started my day with yoga and meditation, feeling refreshed like never before.

That experience changed my perspective. I understood that even though I had managed my time well before, there was another level of peace and clarity that could be reached. It made me realize how much healing there is in slowing down. Now, I strive to incorporate more moments of slow, intentional living into my daily routine.

How to Slow Down

Slowing down doesn't mean stepping away from life; it means engaging with it more fully. Here are some ways to cultivate a SlowFlow lifestyle:

- **Relish your coffee or tea:** Savour each sip. Allow warmth to ground you, and notice the aroma, the taste and the experience of each moment.
- **Eat with gratitude:** Instead of rushing through meals, take time to appreciate the food on your plate. Be grateful for the nourishment it provides.
- **Connect with nature:** Spend time outdoors. Listen to the rustling leaves, feel the wind on your skin and let nature slow your racing mind.
- **Pause with loved ones:** Don't rush your interactions. Whether it's with your children, parents or friends, be fully present and enjoy those moments.
- **Unplug regularly:** Designate screen-free times. Turn off devices and focus on activities that feed your soul—reading, creating art or simply being.
- **Single-tasking:** Shift from multitasking to single-tasking. Focus on completing one task at a time, giving it your full attention. Start with simple tasks like eating without checking your phone or listening to music without doing other activities.
- **Engage in slow hobbies:** Activities like knitting, painting or gardening are naturally slow and repetitive, helping to calm the nervous system. These hobbies allow you to immerse yourself in the present, finding rhythm in the slowness.
- **Slow down your breathing:** Practise slow, deep breathing, such as the 4–7–8 technique (inhale for 4 counts, hold for 7 and exhale for 8).

- **Cook or bake from scratch:** Cooking or baking is a great way to slow down, as it requires attention to the process. It encourages mindfulness through chopping, stirring and measuring.
- **Create a morning or evening ritual:** Establish a ritual that signals the beginning or end of the day, such as lighting a candle, reading a few pages of a book or drinking herbal tea.

Moreover, studies have shown that people who regularly practise slowing down, through activities like yoga, Tai Chi or simple, mindful walks, have lower levels of inflammation in their bodies. This is significant because chronic inflammation is linked to a host of age-related diseases, from cardiovascular issues to cognitive decline.

The practice of slowing down is not about doing less but about doing better—living better. We can achieve our goals, reach new heights and still maintain a sense of inner peace.

Slow down, even if it's for a few minutes.

42

Intimacy, Lovemaking, Orgasms and the Afterglow

The process of arousal, lovemaking and afterglow involve a beautiful balance of both the sympathetic and parasympathetic states for a fulfilling experience. The SNS provides excitement and energy, while the PNS brings calm and connection. When our body is in harmony, it can shift seamlessly between these states. An imbalance—such as chronic stress or heightened anxiety—can disrupt this flow, making it difficult to enjoy intimacy.

Understanding the Nervous System: Sympathetic and Parasympathetic Interplay

During arousal, the body initially leans on the SNS to build excitement, and as we progress through foreplay to orgasm, the PNS begins to take on the reins, promoting relaxation and connection.

Arousal: The Starting Point

Arousal is the starting point of intimacy. It's not just about the body, but also about the mind. Emotional connection, anticipation and desire all play a role in this stage. When we experience arousal, our bodies release adrenaline and norepinephrine, causing the heart to race, blood flow to increase towards the genitals and our senses to heighten.

- **Sympathetic Activation:** At the beginning, the sympathetic nervous system takes charge. This explains the quickened heartbeat, dilated pupils and increased breathing rate—your body is literally 'excited'. Blood flow increases, preparing the body for pleasure.
- **Mental Arousal:** The brain, our most powerful sex organ, is the key here. The release of dopamine—a neurotransmitter linked to pleasure—enhances desire. Dr Emily Nagoski, author of *Come As You Are*, explains that 'context is everything' when it comes to arousal. The brain creates desire when we feel safe, comfortable and stimulated by our surroundings.

Foreplay: Building Connection and Trust

Foreplay is not just a prelude to sex; it is where intimacy truly deepens. It involves touch, words, eye contact and connection. It allows partners to attune to each other's needs, building a sense of trust and safety, which is critical for shifting from the SNS to the PNS.

- **Sensory Stimulation:** Gentle touches, deep breaths and a slow build-up stimulate the PNS through the vagus nerve, which helps us relax. Foreplay engages all five senses, from touch and sound to smell, helping to deepen emotional connection.
- **Release of Oxytocin:** Known as the 'cuddle hormone', oxytocin is released during touching, kissing and cuddling, creating a bond between partners and promoting feelings of safety. Oxytocin's ability to counteract cortisol makes it an important hormone for stress relief. Studies published in the *Journal of Sexual Medicine* have shown that high levels of oxytocin are

associated with lower stress levels and a heightened sense of well-being.

Orgasm: The Climax of Connection

Orgasm represents a peak moment where the body undergoes a powerful shift between the sympathetic and parasympathetic states.

- **Sympathetic Surge:** At the point of climax, the SNS fires once more, creating intense muscle contractions, elevated heart rate and increased breathing. It's an explosive moment that many describe as a physical and emotional release.
- **The Shift to Parasympathetic:** Immediately after orgasm, the PNS takes over. This is when the body experiences a deep sense of relaxation, often referred to as the 'afterglow'. During this time, dopamine and endorphins flood the brain, creating a sense of pleasure and satisfaction.

Afterglow and Connection: The afterglow is often overlooked, but it holds immense importance. This phase allows oxytocin and serotonin to continue their work, building a sense of connection and peace. A study published on *The Journal of Neuroscience* found that orgasm significantly reduces the activity of the amygdala—the brain's centre for processing fear and anxiety—thereby promoting calm and relaxation.

This stage is when partners can experience deeper bonding and healing. It is encouraged to relax in each other's arms, allowing the body to absorb the feelings of comfort and connection fully. It's a way to prolong the positive effects of neurochemicals, allowing for deep relaxation and improved sleep

Why and How Stress Hinders Intimacy

Stress is a common barrier to experiencing pleasure and intimacy. When the body is stuck in the sympathetic mode due to chronic stress, it becomes difficult to relax enough to enjoy arousal or achieve orgasm. Elevated cortisol levels, the body's primary stress hormone, can interfere with the production of sex hormones, like testosterone and oestrogen, leading to reduced libido and conditions like Erectile Dysfunction or Vaginismus. While the reasons behind these conditions could be multifactorial, stress is a big contributor. A *Journal of Psychosomatic Medicine* study has also highlighted that chronic stress significantly diminishes sexual arousal and pleasure.

Stress can lead to 'spectatoring', a term coined by sex therapists Masters and Johnson, where an individual becomes overly self-conscious during sexual activity, worrying about their performance rather than being in the moment. This anxiety can inhibit the natural flow from SNS to PNS, preventing orgasm and enjoyment.

What if you don't have a partner? Intimacy is not only reserved for those in relationships. Self-love and self-pleasure, including masturbation, can offer similar benefits for regulating the nervous system. It's about tuning into your own body, understanding what feels good and creating a safe space for yourself.

Studies published in *Journal of Sex & Marital Therapy* have shown that masturbation releases similar endorphins and oxytocin, reducing stress and promoting relaxation. When approached mindfully, self-pleasure can be a way to explore your body and understand what brings you comfort and joy. It's an act of self-care that nurtures body awareness and emotional well-being.

Many sexologists emphasize the importance of embracing self-pleasure without guilt or shame. Dr Laurie Mintz, author of *Becoming Cliterate*, suggests that masturbation is a powerful way to connect with your body's needs and desires. By reducing the stigma around self-pleasure, we can shift our perspective to see it as a natural and healthy way to unwind.

Beyond physical touch, intimacy—emotional closeness, shared laughter and vulnerability—can be just as powerful for our nervous system. Feeling safe and understood by a partner, or even by yourself, allows the PNS to activate more fully. Emotional intimacy creates an environment where the body feels secure enough to let go of tension, making it a cornerstone of fulfilling and satisfying lovemaking.

In our coaching, we encourage partners to explore intimacy before diving into the physical act of lovemaking. Human connection is a fundamental need that creates a sense of safety and security. It's a powerful and natural tool that, when used mindfully and safely, can transform health and relationships.

As the *Kama Sutra*, the ancient guide on love and connection, beautifully suggests, 'A person should learn to enjoy themselves and their partner, for that is the true essence of pleasure.' This wisdom teaches us that intimacy is not merely a physical act but a spiritual and emotional connection that can elevate our experience of the world.

43

Practising Smiling

In a world where stress, anxiety and overwhelming responsibilities seem to surround us daily, amongst the several tools we have to manage stress, smiling—yes, a simple, genuine smile—holds more power than we often realize. A smile can down-regulate an up-regulated nervous system, helping us shift from a state of 'fight-or-flight' (sympathetic mode) to 'rest-and-digest' (parasympathetic mode). But why is this so, and how does something as effortless as smiling influence our nervous system and reduce stress?

The Science of Smiling

Every time you smile, whether genuinely or even when faked, you activate certain facial muscles that signal to the brain that all is well. The act of smiling sends messages to the brain that interpret these facial movements as indicators of safety and relaxation. Dr Sarah Pressman, a psychologist specializing in stress research, explains that even the simple act of holding a smile can shift our nervous system towards a parasympathetic state, easing tension and lowering stress hormones.

When we smile, several physiological processes take place:

1. **Activation of the PNS:** Smiling activates the vagus nerve, a major component of the parasympathetic system, which helps down-regulate stress responses, slowing down heart rate and inducing a state of relaxation.
2. **Release of Neurotransmitters:** Endorphins and serotonin, often referred to as 'feel-good' hormones, are released, enhancing our sense of well-being. These neurochemicals not only boost our mood, but also combat stress-related hormones like cortisol and adrenaline.
3. **Increased Blood Flow:** Smiling can increase blood flow to the brain, supporting its healthy functioning and further reducing anxiety levels. Enhanced blood flow helps keep the brain oxygenated and alert, promoting clearer thinking and better emotional regulation.

The Fake Smile: Tricking the Brain into Believing in Calmness

A common question is, 'What if there's nothing to smile about?' Life can sometimes feel overwhelming and finding a reason to smile might seem impossible. This is where the concept of the 'fake smile' comes in—a strategy even leading therapists recommend.

Dr Tara Well, a professor of psychology at Columbia University, emphasizes that the body doesn't always distinguish between a genuine smile and a fake one. By simply activating the muscles involved in smiling, you can influence your brain's interpretation of the environment, helping you feel safer and more relaxed.

In our coaching practice, we often encourage clients to 'fake it till they make it'. Just by smiling, even when you don't feel like it, you send a powerful message to your brain: I'm okay, I'm safe. Clients who were initially sceptical found themselves feeling lighter, as their brain responded to the smile with a cascade of calming reactions. Through repetition, a fake smile can become genuine, transforming a challenging mood into a more positive one.

Even for many of our clients, smiling amidst pain or adversity feels daunting. But in neuroscience, there's a fascinating concept called the 'facial feedback hypothesis', which posits that our facial expressions influence our emotions. Research from NCBI and studies by Dr Paul Ekman, a pioneer in emotion research, show that the act of smiling, even when we don't necessarily feel happy, activates the neural pathways associated with positive feelings.

Imagine a client who has experienced a series of life setbacks, struggling to find a reason to smile. Through guided sessions, we encourage them to practise smiling as a physical exercise, a gentle reminder to their brain that safety and calm are accessible even in tough times. Many report feeling an unexplainable lightness and resilience they didn't expect, all because they practised a simple smile.

Psychologists and medical professionals have taken a keen interest in the effects of smiling on mental health:

- Dr Laura Kubzansky, a professor at Harvard T.H. Chan School of Public Health, points out that positive emotions, like those generated by smiling, can promote cardiovascular health. Her research shows that individuals who smile often tend to have lower blood pressure and reduced risk of chronic stress.
- Dr Martin Seligman, often called the father of positive psychology, underscores that simple actions, such as smiling, can help rewire the brain towards optimism, supporting long-term emotional health.
- Even the APA highlights smiling as a 'simple but profound tool' for emotional regulation. In moments of high stress, the APA recommends techniques like mindful smiling, which pairs the act of smiling with breathing to promote relaxation and grounding.

Incorporating smiling into your daily life is simpler than it might seem. Here are a few ways to start:

1. **Set a Reminder to Smile:** Start with small moments. Set a gentle reminder on your phone to smile for a few seconds, every hour, especially during stressful times.
2. **Mindful Smiling Exercise:** Try a practice of mindful smiling each morning. Smile gently as you breathe deeply, holding the smile for a few seconds with each breath.
3. **Smile to Relax Muscles:** When you feel tension creeping in, take a moment to pause and smile. This act can instantly signal your body to relax muscles, easing stiffness in the neck, face and shoulders.
4. **Mirror Practice:** Stand in front of a mirror and smile at yourself. It may feel awkward, but this practice helps reinforce the feeling of safety and well-being, and can make smiles feel more genuine over time.

Smiling is a potent, underrated tool for managing stress and balancing our nervous system. The next time you find yourself overwhelmed, try smiling. It might feel forced at first, but remember that even a fake smile signals your brain to create positive feelings. You're not just changing your facial expression; you're actively down-regulating your nervous system and creating a space of calmness.

In the words of Dr Pressman, 'A smile isn't just a response; it's a pathway to feeling better, one small step at a time.' So, practise smiling. Let it become a small act of self-care, a signal to your brain that calm, joy and resilience are within reach.

44

Bonfire/Sitting by a Fireplace

Ever wondered why sitting by a campfire feels so deeply satisfying? The crackle of wood, the warm glow and the comforting heat against the cold air . . .

The magic of a bonfire goes beyond just the physical warmth it offers; it taps into something ancient within us, providing a powerful way to relax and regulate our nervous systems.

For our ancestors, fire was more than warmth; it was safety, community and survival. The presence of a controlled fire meant protection from predators, warmth in harsh climates and the ability to cook food. Fire gatherings became social rituals, allowing early humans to form bonds, share stories and feel secure. The crackling of fire, in particular, signalled a safe environment, reassuring the nervous system and allowing for rest. Sitting around a fire, our ancestors would feel secure, allowing their nervous systems to regulate from the heightened vigilance required for survival. The warmth of the fire would soothe muscles, and the visual effect of the flames' rhythmic movement could even induce a meditative state.

In today's world, that same sense of security and relaxation can be felt when we sit by a bonfire or fireplace.

Research has shown that watching the flickering flames of a fire activates our PNS. The rhythmic and mesmerizing movement of flames has a trance-like effect that mimics the relaxation experienced through practices like meditation or yoga. Studies published by NCBI and on PubMed suggest that this visual pattern helps the brain enter a meditative state, thus reducing anxiety, calming the mind and slowing the heart rate.

One study, in particular, observed that individuals who watched a fire showed significant decreases in blood pressure, compared to those who did not. The multi-sensory experience of a fire—its warmth, the smell of burning wood, the visual rhythm of the flames and the crackling sounds—engages several senses simultaneously. This sensory input helps to ground us, pulling us into the present moment and giving our minds rest from racing thoughts and concerns. In fact, psychologists often note that sensory engagement like this is beneficial for reducing anxiety and bringing the body into a balanced state.

Dr Christopher Lynn, an anthropologist at the University of Alabama, conducted research showing that sitting by a fire can reduce blood pressure and enhance relaxation. In his study, participants who watched a fire, especially with the crackling sound included, had a greater reduction in stress markers than those who watched a video of a fire with the sound turned off. The sound of crackling itself triggers feelings of safety and contentment, reminding us, on an unconscious level, of safety and warmth, similar to the cues on which early humans relied to signal that the environment was safe for rest.

Even top psychologists have pointed out that people, who frequently take time to connect with natural elements, including fire, tend to have lower levels of chronic stress. Dr Lisa Feldman Barrett, a leading neuroscientist, has explored how the mind is calmed by natural sights and sounds, and fire, specifically, has a unique effect because it combines warmth with rhythm, both of which signal comfort and safety to our brains.

Experts in nervous system research explain that the warmth of a fire soothes the skin's thermoreceptors, which communicate a sense of comfort to the brain, releasing dopamine, a 'feel-good' neurotransmitter. This release helps switch the nervous system from a sympathetic to a parasympathetic mode, helping the body to relax, restore and recover.

How Firelight Connects Us Socially

Fire has a remarkable ability to build social connections. Historically, fire served as a gathering point for our ancestors, bringing people together to share stories, form alliances and create memories. This communal experience continues to resonate today and sitting by a fire with loved ones can be deeply healing and grounding.

Studies on social bonding have shown that the warmth and light of a fire can increase levels of oxytocin, a hormone associated with bonding, trust and relaxation. In modern psychology, this is sometimes referred to as 'firelight effect', a term used to describe how fire enhances feelings of connection and lowers social barriers. The simple act of gathering around a fire, therefore, helps us connect not only with others but also with ourselves, reducing the feeling of isolation that modern life often brings.

Sitting by a fire is not just an activity; it is a powerful tool for well-being. Here's how it benefits our mind and body:

- **Decreased Stress Levels:** The calming sight and sound of flames lower cortisol levels, which, in turn, reduces feelings of anxiety and stress.
- **Improved Heart Rate and Blood Pressure:** Studies show that being around a fire can help lower heart rate and blood pressure, indicating relaxation and reduced stress.
- **Enhanced Social Bonding:** The warmth of a fire encourages social interactions, which are essential for mental well-being.

- **Improved Sleep Quality:** Spending time around natural elements, including fire, can help regulate circadian rhythms, ultimately improving sleep quality.

For me, the sight of a fireplace on a cold Christmas night is the symbol of comfort. It's almost a family tradition to sit around the fire as we welcome the new year, reflecting on memories and plans for the future. Whether I'm at home or seeking warmth in a log cabin in Finland, a fireplace represents more than just heat.

It's an experience that soothes the soul and brings a grounding stillness, helping me reset and unwind from the world's noise.

45

The Power of Manifestation

Imagine a world where your thoughts act as seeds and your mind is the fertile soil in which they grow. Every thought and intention possess the potential to manifest into outcomes.

Manifestation is not a buzzword. It is more than just wishful thinking, daydreaming or idle wishing. It is the art of harnessing the incredible power of your mind to bring your desires to fruition. I keep talking about manifestation because it works.

How Do You Make Manifestation Work for You?

Manifestation doesn't just mean you can sit on a couch all day and visualize earning a billion dollars, your cancer going into remission or love coming into your life without putting in any effort to make it happen.

How to Master Manifestation in Three Steps

Step 1: Visualize crystal clear. Picture what you want vividly. See it through your mind's eye and make it feel real. The clearer your vision, the stronger the pull towards it.

Step 2: Act as if it has already happened. Feel the emotions of receiving what you desire. Imagine the joy, satisfaction and excitement as if it's already happened. Embody these feelings daily.

Step 3: Surrender the outcome. Focus on your efforts, not the results. Trust that the universe knows what's best for you.

The power of manifestation has gained significant attention in recent years. But it has ancient roots.

- It can be traced back to ancient spiritual and philosophical traditions, particularly in the East. Hindu and Buddhist teachings emphasize the power of intention and mental focus to shape reality. The 'Law of Karma' in Hinduism, for example, proposes that thoughts, words and actions influence one's future reality.
- Ancient Greek and Egyptian teachings, especially the Hermetic texts, describe the concept of mentalism, which suggests that 'the all is mind' and that the universe itself is a mental construct. Hermetic principles from *The Kybalion* (Three Initiates, 1908), rooted in much older teachings, discuss how thoughts create reality, similar to modern manifestation ideas.
- In the late nineteenth century, the New Thought movement popularized the idea of the mind's influence over reality in Western culture. Figures like Phineas Quimby, William James and later, Napoleon Hill, contributed to the concept that positive thinking and visualization could lead to desired outcomes. Hill's seminal work, *Think and Grow Rich* (1937), encouraged readers to focus on goals with unwavering belief, a cornerstone of manifestation practices today.
- Rhonda Byrne's *The Secret* (2006) brought the Law of Attraction into mainstream culture, building on previous works by author and father of positive thinking, Norman Vincent Peale. This philosophy suggests that your thoughts are directly linked to what you attract in life, encouraging people to visualize success and focus on positive emotions to manifest their goals.

What Does Science Say?

- Manifestation isn't just about sitting back and visualizing your dream life—it's about doing the work too. Gabriele Oettingen's chapter titled 'Positive Fantasy and Motivation' in the book *The Psychology of Action: Linking Cognition and Motivation to Behavior* (1996) shows that while imagining a great future can feel good, it can actually lower your motivation if it's not backed by action. Why? Because your brain starts to feel like you've already achieved the goal, it relaxes instead of gearing up to chase it. This is why just visualizing success isn't enough. You've got to follow it up with clear steps, real effort, and a plan to overcome obstacles. So yes, dream big—but don't stop there. The magic really happens when you combine belief with bold action.
- A study in *Psychosomatic Medicine* found that optimistic individuals had better immune function and cardiovascular health (Boehm et al., 2020). While this doesn't directly prove the concept of manifestation, it aligns with the theory that a positive mindset can lead to tangible benefits.
- Studies on mindfulness and cognitive reframing, such as one published in the *Journal of Anxiety Disorders* show that actively shifting thoughts can reduce anxiety and depression, and improve overall resilience, especially among those with social anxiety disorders (Shikatani et al., 2014).
- The Reticular Activating System (RAS) is a part of the brain that filters information based on what we deem important (Posner and Petersen, 1990). Neuroscientists suggest that focusing intently on specific goals or outcomes may prime the brain to notice related opportunities, an effect that may underlie the power of manifestation.

What if Your Manifestation Fails?

If a manifestation doesn't materialize, it wasn't meant for you. Trust that you're being protected and guided towards something greater.

Reflections from My Own Life

My life is built on manifestation and visualization. Over the last ten to fifteen years, everything I wanted at a particular time, I have received most of it. However, I've also faced failures, which, in hindsight, were blessings. Trust the universe— it knows what's best for you.

How to Make Manifestation Effective

- **Operate from abundance, hope, faith and belief, instead of a space of lacking, fear and insecurity:** Instead of thinking, 'I don't have money or a job. How can I feel abundant?' tell yourself, 'I believe that I am worthy of getting that job, getting that love, getting that abundance. I am worthy of my disease going away.' There is a big difference between operating from two spaces. When we operate from a space of lacking, we feel we are not worthy enough to get something. We are insecure and fearful. These are very low energies. When we operate from a low-energy space, we only attract things and people at that particular energy and frequency. It is what the law of attraction, quantum physics and the power of the subconscious mind teach us. But what happens when we start operating from a space of abundance? Everything changes.
- **Give up the crab mentality:** If you ever go to the fish market, look into a bucket of live crabs. You will observe this. Each crab is trying to push down the other crabs in a bid to climb out of the bucket. This is called the crab mentality—when people are not happy

with other people's success. They live with envy and try to pull others down. When someone is promoted or rich, they immediately try to find negatives instead of wishing them success. A classic example is how the richest people have the most trolls. Why do we engage in crab mentality? It is because we don't feel good about ourselves. When we project our negativity onto them, we try to feel better and more important. You will not be successful by pulling down other people. The trolls that hide behind a keyboard or live in plain sight among us will always be trolls. Their lives don't change. They can never attract success because they operate from a negative space. If you want to feel successful, start wishing success for the people around you.

- **Wish well for others:** Your thoughts influence your reality. Wishing success and happiness for others opens the flow of positive energy into your own life. I had a patient who said, 'Luke, I was sitting among sixteen other patients going through chemotherapy and forgot my pain. All I did was pray that all those people getting chemotherapy may get better, may not suffer through side effects and that they get into remission.' Beautiful, right? Whatever you want in your life—health, abundance or success—start wishing it for other people.
- **Forgive and release negativity:** Holding onto bitterness and resentment blocks your manifestations. Wish peace for those who hurt you to release these negative energies. It is easier said than done. No one said it was easy. But no one said it was impossible either. One of the best ways out of the numerous techniques for forgiveness is to start feeling good for the person who hurt you. Yes, the hurt may run deep. But you are not doing this for them. You are doing this for your own peace. Right now, you may have thoughts of revenge. All of us go through these feelings. I go through them

when cheated in the company or business. I think of revenge. Soon, however, I realize how bitter I am when the energies around me change. I start attracting the wrong people and events. It is when I tell myself, 'You have felt your feelings of revenge. It is okay. Now, wish them well and move on.' The moment I make that shift, new opportunities start coming into my life. All of a sudden, I realize that I had to lose that business to build a better one. I had to lose that patient with attitude issues to get ten better patients who respect my work and genuinely need me. That is the beauty of abundance and manifestation. It all comes down to introspection.

Drop the Entitlement

We think life should always be easy. That we are entitled to a great life. Drop that entitlement. Sure, we can wish for a good life. But it will never be a bed of roses. It comes with happiness and sadness, wins and defeats. However, the point is to keep moving. You may think, 'Should I wish success for those who do it the wrong way, too?' Karma will fall into place for them. It is for life to decide, not you. Your judgement and opinions don't change anything.

A Life Lesson

We tend to become self-centred and think only about our suffering, negativity, hurt and betrayal. We often forget that there is someone suffering and hurting more than we are.

I want to share a powerful incident from my own life. My dad passed away a couple of years ago. When I visited the graveyard where we had buried him, I stood there in sadness, shock and grief. I looked to the side and saw a picture of a young girl buried at the tender age of twelve.

Something shifted in me. I walked around the cemetery and looked at all the children buried there. Right then, my suffering melted. I was still sad but I realized that someone out there is suffering worse than I am. I found my peace and healing.

You Are the Creator of Your Own Energies

Start creating beautiful energies. Who can do this? Not your religious leader, doctor or nutritionist. You create these energies with how you think and feel.

I had a patient who had back pain. He went in for a back surgery and never got off the table. He is in a wheelchair. Now, the point is: how do we search for compassion for something like this? All we can do is just start a simple prayer every morning for every doctor, neurosurgeon or healthcare practitioner. We pray that they have the power and the courage to do the right thing and be guided the right way. That's how we send out great energies into the world.

It is our way of releasing the shackles, which hold us down, of bitterness, resentment or negativity. If you have been wishing the exact opposite for others and wishing for bad things to happen, you need to stop. We block our abundance because of the negative energies we create.

Manifestation does not mean we can get lazy, greedy and complacent, and expect everything to happen for us. Hard work, talent, discipline, consistency and moving to action are crucial. Drop the entitlement, embrace the journey and trust the process.

46

Praying and Wishing Others Well

Wish well for someone who has hurt you or let you down. Wish for them all what you would wish for your loved ones. Do this as often as you can. It might sound counterintuitive, but it can be one of the most transformative acts of kindness—both towards them and towards yourself. Slowly and steadily, with practice, feel the magic of an energy shift.

Why Does This Matter? A Science-Backed Perspective

When you send positive thoughts or pray for someone who has hurt you, your body's stress response decreases. Studies link forgiveness to a range of health benefits, from lower blood pressure to improved immune function. Dr Frederic Luskin, director of the Stanford Forgiveness Projects, in his book, *Forgive for Good: A Proven Prescription for Health and Happiness* (2002) writes how people who cultivate forgiveness show increased hopefulness, lower stress and reduced symptoms of depression. Wishing someone well—even in small ways—reduces our physiological response to stress and lowers cortisol, which can positively impact heart health and reduce the risk of chronic disease.

Forgiveness and benevolent thinking also affect brain health. A study published in *Social Cognitive and Affective Neuroscience* found that when people engage in compassionate thinking, they activate the brain's reward system (Klimecki et al., 2014). In other words, when we think positively about someone—even if they have wronged us—we activate the same reward centres associated with connection and joy. This helps lift us out of anger and bitterness, emotions that can fuel physical ailments over time.

Forgiveness benefits the heart, literally. A study published in the *Journal of Behavioral Medicine* found that people who practise forgiveness have lower blood pressure and heart rates, leading to improved cardiovascular health (Lawler et al., 2003).

The Healing Magic of Letting Go

Holding onto negative emotions, like resentment and anger, is like carrying an invisible weight. Over time, this weight can manifest into physical symptoms—muscle tension, chronic fatigue and even digestive issues. The mind and body are profoundly connected, and unresolved emotional tension can lead to inflammation, often called the silent killer in medical research. By releasing these emotions, we not only find mental clarity but can also ease our physical burdens.

When we practise forgiveness, we also strengthen our resilience, which allows us to let go of harmful thoughts more easily in the future. By letting go of grudges, we experience a sense of freedom, a new openness to peace, and a renewed connection to others and ourselves.

Traditional Practices of Benevolence

Cultures around the world have long recognized the healing power of forgiveness. In many Buddhist traditions, practitioners engage in *Metta Bhavana,* or loving-kindness meditation, which involves sending love and goodwill to oneself, loved ones, strangers and finally to those with whom we have difficulties. This builds empathy, compassion and resilience, helping practitioners to see beyond their hurt.

Similarly, many indigenous traditions include forgiveness and empathy rituals, especially during community gatherings, where people sit in circles and share grievances, later offering kind words to those who hurt them. This collective release allows for mutual healing, showing the power of community in creating forgiveness and empathy.

How Do We Do This?

1. **Start small.** Begin by wishing well for someone who has only slightly hurt or disappointed you—perhaps, a friend who let you down or a colleague who annoyed you. Imagine them being happy and at peace, and wish for their well-being. Gradually, work your way up to those who have caused deeper pain. Repeat this until it feels less difficult.
2. **Consistency is key.** Make this a regular practice. Set aside a few minutes each day, perhaps during your morning routine or before bed, to send positive thoughts or prayers to someone who has hurt you. You don't need to forgive right away; just start with well-wishing.
3. **Add visualization to this practice.** Focus on your breathing and imagine sending love and good wishes to the person who hurt you. When you feel relaxed, picture the person who hurt you. Visualize them in a peaceful, happy state, free from pain or anger. Imagine a warm light around them, wishing them well-being and healing. This simple exercise can be emotionally intense but is incredibly freeing.
4. **Write about the person who hurt you,** exploring their possible motivations, struggles and humanity. By writing, you acknowledge your feelings but also practise seeing from their perspective. This promotes empathy and lets you release some of the hurt.
5. **Write a compassionate letter to the person who hurt you.** Do not send this. Express your feelings honestly

but end with well-wishing. 'May you find peace. May you find healing.' Keep this letter for yourself, as a symbol of your ability to forgive.

When you wish well for those who have hurt you, you build a muscle of compassion. This practice opens you up to deeper connections with others, teaching you to view pain with a wider lens, and approach relationships with empathy and understanding.

The next time someone hurts you, remind yourself of this: forgiveness is a gift you give to yourself. It's a step towards healing. This isn't about condoning harmful behaviour or ignoring hurt. It's about choosing to release bitterness and wishing peace for others so that you can find peace within yourself. It is an act of strength and courage. It doesn't cost you money. It may be difficult. But difficult doesn't mean impossible. Practise. Practise. And practise.

47

Yawning

Did you always think only bored, tired or sleepy people yawn? You are in for a surprise. What if we told you that yawning could help activate your PNS?

The Science of Yawning

Try yawning as you read this. Do you notice how it involves a deep breathing pattern? You start with a deep inhale followed by a slower exhale. It helps stimulate your vagus nerve, promotes relaxation and even lowers stress levels!

Research published in *Physiology and Behavior* indicates that the act of yawning increases blood flow to the brain and facilitates the exchange of cooler air, which can help regulate brain temperature (Gallup and Gallup, 2008).

A Cooler Brain = A More Efficient and Calm Brain

When you yawn, you take in a large amount of air, which increases oxygen intake. A study published in *Frontiers of Evolutionary Neuroscience* found that yawning enhances the exchange of oxygen and carbon dioxide, leading to improved oxygenation of the brain (Corey et al., 2012).

Better Oxygenation = Enhanced Alertness and Cognitive Function

Yawning helps stretch facial muscles and sometimes even the upper body, if accompanied by stretching your limbs. It releases physical tension and promotes relaxation. It is often a part of the body's natural relaxation response, which reduces heart rate, lowers blood pressure and helps your body shift from heightened alertness to a more relaxed state.

How to Practise Intentional Yawning

- Try yawning intentionally, especially in stressful moments. Take deep, slow breaths and stretch your mouth wide open, mimicking a natural yawn. Focus on how it feels as you stretch your facial muscles.
- Pair your intentional yawning with deep diaphragmatic breathing exercises to enhance the relaxation response. Inhale deeply through your nose, allowing your abdomen to expand fully, and then exhale slowly through your mouth. Repeat this several times to maximize relaxation.
- While yawning, incorporate gentle stretches for your arms, neck and shoulders. Raise your arms above your head, stretch your neck side to side and roll your shoulders back. This combination helps release tension and promotes a feeling of calmness.

In some cultures, yawning is believed to signify a transition from one state of consciousness to another. In certain Indigenous practices, yawning is viewed as a way to invite good energy and dispel negative energy.

The next time you feel the urge to yawn, don't suppress it—embrace it! Yawning is not just a sign of boredom; it's a powerful, natural response that can enhance your mental clarity, regulate your emotions and promote physical well-being. So, go ahead, take a deep breath and let that yawn flow.

48

Mindful Body Scan

Mindful body scanning is a powerful mindfulness practice where you systematically focus attention from your head to toe and progressively relax every muscle. It encourages deep relaxation and heightened awareness of bodily sensations.

The Science Behind Mindful Body Scanning

Beyond decreased levels of stress and anxiety, a study in the *Annals of the New York Academy of Sciences* indicated that mindfulness practices could enhance sleep quality and reduce insomnia symptoms (Rusch et al., 2019). Participants, who engaged in mindfulness meditation, including body scanning, reported better sleep patterns and increased feelings of restfulness.

Research published in the *Journal of Behavioral Medicine* highlighted that body scanning can enhance interoceptive awareness—the ability to perceive internal bodily signals (Ussher et al., 2014). This increased awareness can lead to better emotional regulation and coping strategies.

How to Do It?

Here's a step-by-step guide:

1. Sit or lie down comfortably in a quiet place where you won't be disturbed. Close your eyes to improve your focus.

2. Bring your awareness to your breath first. This sets the stage for the body scan.
3. Slowly direct your attention to each of your body parts, one by one. Start from the top of your head and move towards the toe. The key is to move gradually, focusing on each area, without judgement.
4. As you do this, notice any sensations you feel there—tingling, warmth, coolness, tension, relaxation or any other feeling.
5. Notice any tension in your forehead or jaw? Allow it to soften. Feel for any tightness and breathe into those areas.
6. Observe sensations in your arms, wrists and fingers. Let it go.
7. Tune into your breath and any sensations in your chest and abdomen areas, allowing them to expand and relax.
8. Notice any areas of discomfort in your back? Breathe into them.
9. As you move down, feel the weight of your legs and the contact of your feet with the ground. Imagine your breath bringing relaxation and ease into every spot.
10. By focusing on each body part with curiosity and non-judgement, you activate the PNS.
11. Once you've scanned your entire body, take a moment to appreciate the calmness and awareness you've cultivated. Slowly bring your awareness back to the room, opening your eyes when you're ready.

Practise this well. It helps you develop greater awareness of your body and its signals, encourages relaxation and reduces stress by shifting your focus away from anxious thoughts and into the physical sensations of the present moment.

You can enhance this practice further by using guided meditation apps or breath counting. We will discuss some of the beautiful practices in our upcoming chapters. Keep an eye out.

49

Morning Routines

What is the first thing you do when you wake up in the morning? Is it reaching out to your phone and being overstimulated with a load of messages and notifications? If you are nodding your head affirmatively as you read this, you need to stop. What you need, instead, is to build a solid morning routine.

Why Should You Build a Solid Morning Routine?

Think of your morning as the most sacred hour of the day. How you wake up feeling and what you do in that initial hour can decide the direction of the rest of your day.

What happens when you use your phone first thing when you wake up?

Your brain has billions of neurons, which connect and communicate with each other through tiny electrical currents that travel through them and the enormous networks they form. When all these neurons are activated, they produce electrical pulses. This synchronized activity results in a brainwave.

One of the four primary brainwaves is the alpha state. It is where you are almost awake, physically. It is a state of accelerated learning, relaxed awareness and unconscious absorption of information. When you wake up, your mind is in the alpha state. Any suggestion you make to yourself (affirmations or thoughts—positive or negative) is taken up and imprinted by your brain. When you use this state to check your phone, first thing in the morning, you rewire your brain to reduce productivity and affect how you feel or behave all day long. You rewire your brain to be highly distracted. Your brain starts releasing dopamine, and your nervous system goes into overdrive with every like, share and comment.

You also train your mind to be reactive. You wake up in a highly relaxed state of awareness, but the minute you see bad news, an angry text message or an email that stresses you out, you are in a bad mood for the rest of the day. You are impressionable and almost in a hypnotic state upon waking. You cannot be in control of your day when you are constantly reacting to every situation around you.

This is why we coach our clients to avoid the use of phones and scrolling social media for at least 1 hour after waking up.

The Science Behind Morning Routines

- Research has shown that a structured morning routine can significantly influence mental health. A study published in the *American Journal of Lifestyle Medicine* found that having a consistent morning routine could lower levels of anxiety and improve overall mood (Arlinghaus and Johnston, 2018). Establishing a predictable pattern could help reduce the stress of decision-making, leading to better mental clarity.
- According to a study in the *Journal of Applied Social Psychology*, individuals who follow a structured morning routine are more productive throughout the day (Kirby and Kirby, 2006). Morning rituals help prime the mind for a productive day by creating a sense of control and direction.
- Research published in the *Journal of Behavioral Medicine* shows that individuals who exercise in the morning are more likely to stick to their fitness

goals compared to those who exercise later in the day (Brooker et al., 2023).

Getting Inspired By Our Ancestors and the Armed Forces

Many ancient cultures recognized the importance of starting the day intentionally. The Egyptians had a daily ritual that included prayers and meditation to connect with the divine, setting a positive tone for the day ahead. Even in India, it's a common practice to begin your day with gratitude, having a bath and morning prayer.

In Japan, the practice of *asa-zumi* (morning dew) involves waking up early to perform quiet, reflective tasks, such as tea preparation or garden tending.

Morning routines hold particular significance in military training and operations too.

- The armed forces emphasize the importance of a structured morning routine to instil discipline and promote mental readiness. Early morning exercises and drills are a staple of military life for camaraderie and physical fitness. A report from the *U.S. Army Research Institute for Behavioral and Social Sciences* (Gade et al., 2006) indicates that this structured start can enhance soldiers' resilience and focus.
- In many military units, morning routines often include team-building exercises, morning briefings or shared meals. These practices help strengthen bonds among team members, to build trust and collaboration.

How Can You Build a Powerful Morning Routine?

You don't need to keep it elaborate or excessive for an hour and a half. You can follow a 10–20-minute morning ritual. However, keep it solid and follow it with discipline and consistency. Here are a few tips:

1. **Your body follows the circadian rhythm.** Having a fixed sleep and wake-up time will help you align with this. This biological clock governs various processes in your body, from how you sleep, eat, digest, and secrete certain hormones, and bowel movements to detoxification, among other functions. Yes, once a week, when you are partying and socializing, it is okay to sleep in the next day. But, for at least five out of seven days, try to maintain a routine.
2. **Poop first thing in the morning.** It helps you clean your system. Get done with nature's call. In most cases, a well-functioning body and digestive system will make you want to wake up and immediately go to the loo to pass a motion. It is normal because when you are asleep, your body undergoes a cleansing process. This is why when you wake up, you have dirt between your eyes, morning breath and a white coat on your tongue (it shouldn't be yellow). It is a sign that your digestion is complete, and all your waste is collected in your large intestine, waiting to be eliminated. That's the beauty of a sleep-wake cycle.
3. **Finish your hygiene routine.** You may do your oil pulling or brush your teeth, get a shave or take a shower. Follow your basic hygiene routine next.
4. **Get that movement.** This can include simple stretches, yoga asanas, pranayama, breathing exercises, running, hitting the gym, or *Tabata*—anything that gets you moving. Being active in the morning can boost your blood circulation, pump your arteries and nourish every cell with the life force—oxygen. It wakes up your immune system and kick-starts your metabolism. Getting adequate movement also helps your mind and body to wake up and release endorphins (happy hormones), which help you stay positive and approach the day head-on.
5. **Set your intention for the day.** It may seem very airy-fairy to you, but setting intentions is powerful. It sets

the tone for your day. Most people wake up and just respond to life by reacting. But when you have your intention, you set a purpose for your day to follow. When you do not set an intention, your day can spiral into chaos, leading to you missing out on the most important things you need to do for self-care. It takes you 2 minutes or less. Ask yourself: **What is it that I want to accomplish?** Make it crystal clear. When it is registered in your subconscious, there is a very good chance it will materialize in your day. Remember, setting intentions is very different from making a to-do list.

6. **Make your to-do list (try to do this the night before).** Not having a to-do list can make you feel anxious and stressed because you may constantly worry about forgetting important tasks. We usually suggest most of our clients make this to-do list the night before. It helps you plan your day better and takes less than 5 to 10 minutes. Your mind is often cluttered with several thoughts; putting your tasks on a piece of paper can help bring some order and organization to your day. And do not forget to keep striking off the things you accomplished from that list because that can be very rewarding.
7. **Pray if you can.** It is powerful. It is a beautiful tool. It doesn't matter if you are praying to God or the Universe, whether you are sending energy or asking for help. Prayer can be a powerful practice for your well-being and healing. Unfortunately, it is much underutilized. Most people don't pray with faith and belief, which is why many prayers go unanswered. So, place your complete trust and pray deeply. You are now ready to begin the rest of your day. The idea is not to rush but to follow a ritual so that you can unfold the rest of your chores or work for the day calmly with good energy and positivity. Think of it like athletes preparing themselves for a 100-metre

race. There is always preparation before a big event. For you, your morning rituals are a preparation for your big event—the day.

Now, go and conquer your day.

50

The Gift of Deep Sleep

During the COVID-19 lockdown, I was privileged to be nominated by our Hon. Prime Minister Narendra Modi's Fit India Movement as its Wellness Champion and Lifestyle Ambassador. Over the last year, I took on the avatar of Mr Sleep and started recruiting Sleep Angels within my community to promote, encourage and inspire all generations to sleep deeper. Why? Through my practice, over the last thirteen years, I have directly witnessed a link between sleep deprivation and every single disease and condition—physical, mental or emotional. While the world and country are chasing more diet and exercise trends, what about sleep and emotional wellness, which are at the top of the health paradigm? From workplace stress deaths, marathon deaths and young people dropping dead, we can blame many things, but how about looking at sleep?

Deep sleep is very close to my heart because it plays a pivotal role in prevention, healing, energy and being able to enjoy life and feel joyful. Sleep has always been my lynchpin.

I remember the crazy, cheap Mumbai–New York, Mumbai–Belgium and London flights that my clients booked for me, twelve years ago, to fly down and see them, or even me booking the cheapest flights with the longest routes because I couldn't afford it then. The impact all of that had on my sleep was immense. I felt horrible on every level. I had colds, coughs and flu. I couldn't focus mentally, and these flights were almost every one to two months.

I made a personal goal to work hard, smart and so well that, one day, I would be valuable enough and have enough to book my flights and routes around my healthy sleep schedules. My body type needs deep sleep to be my best in my relationships, workouts, work, diagnostic power, planning power and the ability to give my emotions to my sick patients. So, I want to write about sleep and how it is the ultimate calm and reset prescription for the body, brain and soul.

The Calm Prescription: Sleep as the Brain and Body's Magic Restore Button

Sleep is one of the few activities that truly restores and rejuvenates both the brain and the body. It is often referred to as the brain's 'magic restore button' due to its vital role in various physiological, emotional and cognitive functions. Numerous researchers and sleep experts have identified sleep as crucial not only for maintaining health but also for preventing chronic diseases.

Why Sleep Matters

Sleep serves as a foundation for optimal health, offering a myriad of benefits at various levels:

1. **Physical Recovery:** A study in the *Journal of Pediatrics* points out that during sleep, the body repairs tissues, builds bone and muscle and strengthens the immune system. Growth hormone, essential for recovery, is primarily released during deep sleep (slow-wave sleep) (Van Cauter and Plat, 1996).
2. **Emotional Regulation:** Quality sleep is paramount for emotional health. Studies in *Cognitive Therapy and Research* show that insufficient sleep is linked to mood disorders such as depression and anxiety (Hofmann et al., 2012). During REM sleep, the brain processes emotions, allowing for emotional resilience.

3. **Cognitive Functioning:** Sleep enhances memory consolidation, creativity and problem-solving skills. Studies in *Nature Reviews Neuroscience* show that individuals perform better on cognitive tasks when well-rested (Diekelmann and Born, 2010).
4. **Prevention of Chronic Diseases:** Poor sleep is directly correlated with various health issues:
   - Studies by the *Journal of the National Cancer Institute* have shown a significant association between sleep deprivation and increased breast cancer risk (Travis et al., 2016).
   - Another study in the *Journal of Applied Physiology* shows how sleep loss can lead to insulin resistance, a precursor for type-2 diabetes (Spiegel et al., 2005).
   - Inadequate sleep disrupts hormonal balance, leading to increased hunger and cravings, particularly for unhealthy foods, points out a study in *Nature Communications* (Greer, Goldstein, and Walker, 2013).

Stages of Sleep: Understanding the Cycle

Sleep consists of different stages, each vital for various functions. Understanding these stages helps us appreciate why quality sleep is more impactful than merely the quantity.

1. **Non-REM Sleep:**
   - **Stage 1 (Alpha Waves):** This is the lightest stage of sleep, lasting several minutes. You transition from wakefulness, and your breathing and heart rate begin to slow.
   - **Stage 2 (Light Sleep):** Lasting about 20 minutes, this stage features a drop in temperature and slower brainwaves. It is crucial for memory consolidation.
   - **Stage 3 (Slow-Wave Sleep/Delta Waves):** Often referred to as deep sleep, this stage is critical for physical restoration. Blood flow to muscles

increases, and growth hormone is released. This is when the body repairs tissues and strengthens the immune system.

2. **REM Sleep:**
   Rapid eye movement (REM) sleep typically occurs about 90 minutes after falling asleep and constitutes about 25 per cent of total sleep time. During REM, the brain is highly active, and dreams occur. This stage enhances memory and emotional processing, making it vital for overall cognitive functioning, shares British author, scientist and professor of Neuroscience and Psychology, Matthew Walker, in his book *Why We Sleep: Unlocking the Power of Sleep and Dreams* (2017).

The Importance of Quality over Quantity

While the general recommendation is 7–9 hours of sleep per night, for adults, the quality of that sleep is equally, if not more, crucial. Quality sleep encompasses uninterrupted cycles through the different stages, allowing the body to gain restorative benefits.

Lifestyle Changes to Improve Sleep Quality

Implementing certain lifestyle changes can promote deeper sleep and help transition to a more balanced state:

1. **Establish a Sleep Schedule:** Go to bed and wake up at the same time each day to regulate your body's internal clock.
2. **Create a Sleep-Inducing Environment:** Dim the lights as bedtime approaches, ensure a cool room temperature and eliminate noise and distractions.
3. **Limit Electronic Device Exposure:** Blue light emitted by smartphones, tablets and computers can disrupt melatonin production. Try to switch off devices 1–2 hours before bedtime.

4. **Pre-Sleep Routine:** Engage in relaxation techniques, such as reading, meditation or gentle stretches, before bed to help signal your body that it's time to sleep.
5. **Nutrition and Exercise:** Avoid large meals, caffeine and alcohol close to bedtime. Regular physical activity can further improve sleep quality, but ensure workouts are completed early in the day.
6. **Consider Sleep Aids:** While not always necessary, natural supplements like magnesium, melatonin or herbal teas, like chamomile, can support sleep onset.

Always consult a qualified health provider before adding any supplements to your routine.

Tools and Techniques for Deeper Sleep

1. **Meditation and Mindfulness:** These practices can reduce anxiety and improve sleep. A study showed that mindfulness meditation improved sleep quality in participants (*JAMA Internal Medicine*, Black et al., 2015).
2. **Breathwork:** Techniques such as deep breathing can activate the PNS, promoting relaxation and facilitating sleep onset (*Journal of Alternative and Complementary Medicine*, Brown and Gerbarg, 2005).
3. **Nature Sounds and Music:** Calming sounds or soft music can create a soothing atmosphere conducive to sleep (*Journal of Advanced Nursing*, Harmat et al., 2008).
4. **Cognitive Behavioural Therapy for Insomnia (CBT-I):** If sleep issues persist, CBT-I strategies help address underlying disorders and promote healthy sleep habits (*American Journal of Lifestyle Medicine*, Rossman, 2019).

What Are Some More Pre-bedtime Rituals to Help You Fall into Deep Sleep?

- Have early dinners, usually before or close to sunset. As the sun sets, our digestive capacity slows down too. Eating early improves your sleep schedule. It also helps your body carry out the process of digestion with ease. This is how your circadian rhythm works. It also explains why one may wake up feeling heavy, sluggish and lethargic after a late-night heavy meal. This is because your body didn't get a chance to digest and break it down effectively.
- If you can't make it early to your dinners, eat light dinners, at least an hour or two before bedtime.
- Avoid consuming stimulants like tea, coffee, alcohol, spicy foods, tobacco, smoking, social media, news and disturbing conversations around bedtime.
- Solve crossword puzzles, play Sudoku or simply have pleasant conversations with your kids or family members.
- Be consistent with your gadgets and digital cleanse.
- Maintain darker surroundings. Switching off all lights half an hour before bedtime signals the body that it is time for you to fall asleep. Dark rooms also help secrete the sleep hormone, melatonin, otherwise restricted due to artificial lighting.
- Sprinkle or dab essential oils, like lavender, frankincense or vetiver, on your pillow. They are known to promote sleep. You can also use a sleep mist containing these essential oils.
- Try breathing exercises. Close your mouth and right nostril completely. Only use your left nostril to inhale and exhale for a couple of rounds as you lie down to sleep. This calms the body and mind internally, and helps you fall asleep.
- Practice the 4–7–8 breathing technique. Inhale, hold, exhale and repeat for a couple of rounds. Inhale for 4 seconds, hold for 7 seconds and exhale for 8 seconds.

- Read before bedtime. This helps reduce stress, clears the mind and prepares the body to sleep.
- Reflect on your day for a deeper sleep. Close your eyes. Inhale long and slow, then exhale longer than you inhale. Replay your day—how it went, the moments that made you smile. Reflect on what made you feel good about yourself. Acknowledge three things or people you are grateful for. Then, go to sleep.
- Meditate and set intentions. Visualize how you want to spend the next day. Try to maintain a journal where you write it all down before you sleep. Do these at least 10–15 minutes before bedtime. This stops the chatter in your mind, reduces anxiety and helps you sleep peacefully.
- Take a warm shower before bedtime. It provides muscle relaxation and helps you sleep better. You can even add essential oils or Epsom salt in the water to relax your nerves and muscles further.
- Make love. This releases oxytocin, the feel-good hormone, and prolactin, a hormone produced by the pituitary gland. Both of these relax the body and allow you to sleep easily.
- Try yogic practices like *Yoga Nidra* and *Shavasana*. These are quite helpful in sleeping when done close to bedtime.

Having said that, achieving these steps won't happen overnight. Therefore, aim to adopt one ritual at a time. Go for the habit-stacking method. Challenge yourself to eat your last meal early or at least 1–2 hours before bedtime. Stick to it until your body adapts to it gradually. Then, stack the next habit of keeping your gadgets and devices away from your eyesight. Again, the goal is to limit exposure to blue light. If you don't see your gadgets, you are most unlikely to use them. Out of sight is out of mind. Instead, spend that time practising the relaxation activities mentioned above.

When these changes don't feel like a change anymore, stack them with the final habit of sleeping in a completely dark room. Once you have a night routine, stick to it for five out of seven days a week.

With some changes, you can easily adapt these tips to your lifestyle.

Harnessing the Magic of Sleep

Sleep is not merely a period of rest; it is an essential component of our physical, emotional and mental well-being. By prioritizing sleep and implementing lifestyle changes to enhance its quality, we position ourselves to lead healthier, more balanced lives.

As you embark on your journey towards improved sleep, remember that investing in quality rest is one of the most profound forms of self-care you can offer your body and mind—not just in pursuit of calmness but in the quest for overall vitality.

Peaceful, timely and quality sleep is a powerful lifestyle drug. The healing it brings to your body is irreplaceable by any other medication. A good night's sleep is a must to recharge the mind and body. We hope our suggestions will help you abide by a healthy sleeping schedule with simple and effective lifestyle changes. If you are on any kind of sleep medication, please speak to your medical expert before attempting these.

Wish to Try Some Simple Meditations and Visualizations Before Bed?

Scan this QR code for Luke's Guided Meditations.

51

Journalling Your Thoughts and Emotions

This powerful practice holds the potential to transform your life, no matter what situation you may be in. Journalling your thoughts and emotions can help shift your body to switch on the PNS mode.

How?

The act of writing connects the mind and the heart through the pen to a piece of paper. It is crucial for developing neural pathways in our brains.

It helps process and release pent-up emotions, reduces stress, anxiety, and mental clutter and facilitates reflection and a deeper understanding of personal experiences. Besides, this simple exercise requires focus and presence, which makes it incredibly calming and grounding.

The practice of self-reflection through writing dates back centuries. In ancient Egypt, people used hieroglyphics to record their lives and express their emotional and spiritual thoughts. Similarly, the Japanese concept of *shaseibun*—a form of personal essay writing—was used as a reflective tool to capture daily observations and feelings. In ancient Rome, emperors like Marcus Aurelius kept personal journals, which served not only as a record of thoughts but also as a method of cultivating mindfulness and self-awareness.

What Does Science Say?

Beyond managing stress and reducing symptoms of anxiety and depression, journalling can contribute to enhanced cognitive function. Studies published in *Applied Psychology: Health and Well-Being* reveal that consistent writing helps develop neural pathways associated with memory, organization and emotional regulation (Saldanha and Barclay, 2021). This practice also cultivates emotional intelligence by encouraging a deeper understanding of emotions and thought patterns.

Regular journalling can act as a mental cleanse, offering a safe space to release pent-up thoughts and emotions. This practice has been found to support mental clarity and reduce stress by providing a tangible outlet for expressing complex feelings.

Journalling encourages introspection, which can deepen self-understanding and self-compassion. By processing emotions in writing, people can identify triggers and patterns that affect their well-being, giving them the tools to make positive changes.

Research has shown that regular journalling can strengthen the immune system. One study conducted by Dr James Pennebaker, a pioneer in expressive writing research, in the *Journal of Consulting and Clinical Psychology* found that writing about emotional experiences for even 15–20 minutes daily can train immune function by reducing stress and enhancing emotional resilience (Pennebaker, Kiecolt-Glaser, and Glaser, 1988).

Writing down affirmations, expressing gratitude and setting intentions, each day, can help elevate mood and build resilience against life's challenges.

An Exercise for You

Every night, preferably before bed, try this exercise. Clearing your mind before bed can even deepen your sleep quality.

- Find a quiet space where you won't be interrupted.
- Light a candle or play soft music to set the atmosphere.

- Instead of a random notepad, try to use a dedicated journal and a pen that you enjoy writing with.
- Take a few deep breaths and reflect.
- Spend 10–15 minutes writing whatever comes to mind. Don't worry about grammar or structure; just let your thoughts flow.
- Use prompts if needed:
    - What was the best moment of my day?
    - What emotion did I feel most strongly today? What triggered it? How do I respond to it?
    - What am I most grateful for today?
    - What did I learn about myself today?
    - What is my main intention for tomorrow?
- End your journalling with a positive affirmation to seal in the relaxation.

You can also try journalling first thing in the morning, by writing down how you want to feel. For instance, *'Today, I want to feel amazing. I want to feel healthy. I want to feel energetic. I want to be kind.'*

You can do this when you are feeling low, angry or out of control. Open up a page in your journal and start writing anything that comes to mind. It could be the most unhinged thought. It doesn't have to be perfect syntax, punctuation or grammar. Let your thoughts and words flow freely onto the paper. And notice how your feelings shift.

52

Dance Break

In a classic series, revolving around the lives of surgical interns and their supervisors, there's an unforgettable scene. Through the seasons, it makes a comeback in milestone episodes. It's a tradition where the characters process their 'big feelings' with the quirky tradition of 'dancing it out'.

Sounds quirky, right? Only, it is effective.

The Science Behind Dance Breaks

Dance isn't just a joyful activity—it has measurable benefits. Studies in *Frontiers in Psychology* have shown that dancing can significantly increase endorphin levels, creating an instant mood lift and promoting feelings of happiness and relaxation (Koch et al., 2019).

According to research published in *PLOS One,* dance therapy has been found to reduce symptoms of anxiety and depression, while increasing positive mood states (Duarte et al., 2023). Other studies reveal that dance not only improves flexibility and motor skills but also builds social connections and elevates oxytocin or your 'bonding hormone'.

Dancing has been shown to improve HRV, which is an important indicator of overall health and stress resilience. HRV increases when we're relaxed and decreases under stress. Dancing, with its blend of movement, rhythm and emotional expression, acts as a powerful reset, allowing the body to relax while energizing the mind.

Traditional Practices and Ancient Dance Rituals

Dance, as a form of emotional expression and stress relief, is not new. Ancient cultures used dance in ceremonies, often to heal or celebrate life's milestones.

In African tribal dances, for instance, rhythmic movements were used in rituals to convey emotions, connect with others and express collective joy or grief. Indigenous communities in Australia, Africa and South America dance during spiritual ceremonies.

Among the many forms of dance that embody this spirit, the *haka* stands out as a representation of cultural identity, strength and community.

The haka is a traditional Māori war dance from New Zealand. It involves vigorous movements, rhythmic chanting and powerful body percussion. Originally performed by Māori warriors before battle, the haka was intended to intimidate opponents, demonstrate strength and prepare the group, mentally and spiritually, for combat.

Over time, it has evolved into a performance art that is celebrated in various contexts, including sports, ceremonies and cultural events. Each tribe *(iwi)* has its own haka, reflecting their unique history, values and beliefs. Through the haka, performers connect with their ancestry, honour their heritage and reaffirm their cultural identity.

Typically performed by a group, it emphasizes teamwork and solidarity. Each movement and facial expression carry meaning, telling a story of bravery, honour or celebration.

In India, the practice of *nritya* (dance) has been considered a sacred art form used to express deep emotions and even connect with the divine.

How Can You Dance Your Way to Better Emotional Health?

Whether you are processing big feelings or not, try to schedule a 5 or 10-minute dance break during your day, ideally during a natural lull in your routine.

The prerequisites?

- Pick upbeat music that makes you want to move.
- Clear a small area so you don't bump into your furniture.
- Bid those inhibitions goodbye. Drop that self-consciousness and start moving to the beat. Let the music guide you.
- Express any emotions through movement. Jump, sway and spin—whatever feels right.
- As your dance session ends, slow down your movements, and take a few moments to stretch and breathe deeply, transitioning back into your routine.

It's a fun and liberating tool. Try this today.

53

A Tech-Free Day

In this digital age, most of us, like our devices, are always 'online'. But the mental fatigue, stress and anxiety that this can cause is often swept under the carpet.

Take a mindful break from always being available with a tech-free day. A tech-free day is more than just a break from screens; it's an opportunity to reconnect with yourself, your surroundings and the people in your life. By embracing this simple practice, you can cultivate a deeper sense of calmness and restore much-needed balance.

What Does Science Say?

- Recent studies published in the *Journal of Behavioral Addictions* indicate that excessive screen time, especially on smartphones and social media, correlates with higher levels of anxiety, depression and stress (Li et al., 2020).
- A study from the *International Journal of Environmental and Public Health* found that taking tech breaks and reducing screen time improves mental well-being, reduces feelings of loneliness and even enhances overall life satisfaction (Brown and Kuss, 2020). The reduction of blue light exposure is another bonus, as blue light from screens can disrupt sleep by suppressing melatonin production. Taking a

day off from screens can allow your body to realign with its natural circadian rhythms, thus promoting restful sleep.

- A tech-free day can also help reduce sensory overload. Constant notifications and digital multitasking put pressure on our cognitive faculties, affecting focus and increasing mental fatigue.
- Studies suggest that even taking short breaks from screens improves cognitive function and allows the brain to recharge. *Proceedings of the 2016 CHI Conference on Human Factors in Computing Systems* show that people, who take regular tech-free days, report enhanced creativity, improved focus and better emotional resilience (Kushlev, Proulx, and Dunn, 2016).

How to Do This

- Start by tracking your tech time. Your smartphone and gadgets will give you an idea of this in the settings menu. You will be surprised at how much time you spend glued to your phone or computer.
- Choose a day when you have minimal obligations that require digital connectivity. Inform friends, family and colleagues of your intention to be offline (in advance).
- Make a list of what is allowed and prohibited. For instance, you might take emergency phone calls but avoid social media, chatting, emails and streaming services.
- Out of sight is out of mind. If possible, remove or hide digital devices from your immediate surroundings to reduce temptation.
- Fill your day with activities that don't involve screens. Dive into a novel, go for a hike, sit in a park, engage in yoga or meditation, try new recipes, do creative projects, meet a friend or family member, play board

games, enjoy a meal together or engage in physical activities like walking, running or workouts.

- Reflect on your experiences and write down how it made you feel.

Many cultures have ritualized days of rest and reflection, such as the Jewish practice of *Shabbat*, where electronic devices are set aside for a day to focus on family, community and spiritual connections. Similarly, the *Uposatha* days in Buddhism are set aside for refraining from worldly activities to meditate, reflect and restore inner peace. In Ayurveda, technology fasts are also recommended as part of *Dina Charya* (daily routine) to build mindfulness and reduce stress.

The Goal: Balance, Not Elimination

A tech-free day is about balance, not about demonizing technology. Breaking tech habits may feel challenging, but gradual and consistent practice will make it easier over time. Embrace this time as a way to reconnect with what truly matters.

54

Practising Advanced Gratitude

In our practice, we constantly speak about the power of gratitude because it helps us move our focus from what we lack to what we have. Sounds contrived at first, right? However, this mental state only grows stronger with daily practice. We have experienced the transformative power of deep gratitude work beautifully for our clients across ages and stages, including end-of-life.

While there are numerous ways to embrace gratitude—saying thank you, writing gratitude notes or letters, journalling, offering thanks before meals or praying—we want to introduce you to something even more powerful.

Advanced Gratitude

How Does This Work?

In this, you move from the present quantum field to the future quantum field and offer thanks in advance.

Advanced gratitude is a transformative practice where you express thankfulness for future events and outcomes as if they have already occurred.

Some examples of these could be:

- Giving thanks in advance for your medical report to show improvement or successful treatment.

- Offering thanks in advance for your business reaching X per cent of future profits.
- Being grateful for the successful completion of a challenging process you are about to start.

Advanced gratitude aligns with the law of attraction, where focusing on positive outcomes helps manifest them.

It makes you grateful for what you have right now and for what the future holds in store for you. You lose nothing by intending for the best.

Science on the Attitude of Gratitude

- A study published in the *Journal of Personality and Social Psychology* found that people who kept a daily gratitude journal experienced a 25 per cent increase in happiness after just ten weeks (Emmons and McCullough, 2003). The simple act of reflecting on things, for which they were grateful, helped reframe their thinking, leading to a more positive outlook on life.
- According to the National Institutes of Health (NIH), gratitude activates brain areas associated with dopamine release, promoting pleasure and motivation. This neurological response makes advanced gratitude an excellent tool for visualizing and reinforcing future goals (Diniz et al., 2023).
- Appreciation also strengthens our ability to cope with adversity. In a study published in *Psychological Science,* participants who practised gratitude showed lower stress responses when faced with difficult situations (Kumar and Epley, 2018).

Many ancient cultures embraced future-focused gratitude as part of their spiritual practices. Native American traditions, for instance, often include thankful prayers for abundant harvests before planting season, expressing gratitude in advance for nature's bounty. Similarly, in *Bhakti Yoga* (a branch of Hindu spiritual practice), practitioners offer gratitude for the realization of future desires, trusting that heartfelt intentions will manifest.

In Japan, *Kan-sha* means sincere gratitude, often expressed through actions rather than words. Japanese people show gratitude in advance through small, intentional actions that honour and respect their goals. You can adapt this by performing an action that symbolizes your future success, like preparing your workspace as if you've already achieved a promotion.

Many Chinese families give thanks in advance for prosperity, health and happiness during the Lunar New Year by offering food and incense to deities, trusting that their wishes will be fulfilled in the coming year.

Exercise to Offer Advanced Gratitude

All you need to do is:

- Spend a few minutes visualizing a future goal or desired outcome.
- Imagine every detail vividly, as if it has already happened.
- Write it down if you can. Start with 'I am grateful for . . .' and describe the future event or outcome in the present tense. For example, 'I am grateful for the promotion I received at work' or 'I am grateful that my blood work parameters are clear.'

Immerse yourself in the emotions of gratitude and joy that come with achieving your goal.

How Can You Deepen This Practice?

Try writing a letter, offering thanks for something that has not yet happened, but you desire. Describe, in detail, the emotions and gratitude you feel for this outcome. Letters offer a physical commitment to the practice, reinforcing your intention.

Practising advanced gratitude regularly conditions your mind to focus on positive possibilities, transforming your mindset and preparing your brain for actualizing those outcomes. With steady practice, you're not just hoping for a brighter future—you're actively inviting it.

55

Staying Present During Your Daily Commute

How often do you feel you are moving on autopilot during your daily commute? Break that monotony. Travelling to work, school, college or any place you need to be, every day, can be taxing for many. Hopping onto that train, cab or bus right in the nick of time can be chaotic, to say the least. But once you do, it can also be the perfect space to practise mindfulness and activate the PNS.

How do you do that? By staying present and immersed in the moment, you can transform your commute from a mundane daily task into a peaceful, grounding, aware and relaxing experience.

How to Start?

- Begin your commute by breathing slowly and deeply. It will signal your body to relax.
- Pay attention to the details of your surroundings, whether you are inside a public transport, driving or walking. Notice the sights, sounds and smells, and engage all your senses—the colour of the buildings, the contrast between light and dark, the trees, the bulletins or the overhead wires running in perfect symmetry. Things you usually wouldn't notice.
- Reflect on and appreciate the ability to commute or the opportunity to see new things along your route.

- Check in with your body. Notice any tension in your muscles and consciously relax them. Pay attention to how your body feels as you move or sit.
- If you're listening to music or a podcast, do so mindfully. Focus on the sounds, lyrics or narration. Let yourself fully immerse in the audio experience.
- Notice the thoughts that arise without being caught up in them. Acknowledge them and gently bring your focus back to the present moment.

Do this well.

The Science Behind Mindful Commuting

- A *Psychoneuroendocrinology* study found that mindfulness practices help reduce cortisol (the stress hormone) levels, which are often high during high-stress moments like rush-hour commutes (Rogerson et al., 2024).
- A *Transportation Research Part F: Traffic Psychology and Behaviour* study found that mindfulness helps commuters stay present, resulting in reduced irritability and improved mood—even in frustrating conditions like delays or traffic jams (LaJeunesse and Rodríguez, 2012).

Making Mindful Commuting a Daily Habit

Over time, regular mindful commuting will help your body and mind associate transit with calmness rather than chaos. Notice how this practice changes your experience of your day, improves patience and reduces commuting fatigue. This small shift from the routine rush to a mindful ritual will not only benefit you on the go but also positively influence your interactions and productivity for the rest of your day.

56

Use Calming Scents/Aromatherapy

Did you know that smell could evoke nostalgia and create a sense of relaxation that is nothing short of magical? Your olfactory system is intimately connected to your brain's limbic system and is a direct pathway to our emotions and memories. This connection explains why certain scents can instantly transport us to cherished moments of the past.

The aroma of food wafting through your home, the scent of freshly baked bread, a simmering pot of soup, cookies just out of the oven or the earthy fragrance of petrichor after the first rain—these remind us of loved ones, childhood, simpler and more carefree times.

A spa, for example, instantly soothes and relaxes you. Besides the ambiance, the fragrance of essential oils brings a sense of calm.

The Science Behind Aromatherapy and Emotional Balance

Scientists have studied the effect of smells on our bodies and minds for the longest time. Studies point out that the ancient practice of aromatherapy can bring about physical, mental and emotional balance.

A study published in *Frontiers in Psychology* demonstrates that smell activates the amygdala and hippocampus, two areas in the brain associated with emotional regulation and memory. This connection allows certain aromas to improve mood and promote relaxation (Larsson et al., 2014).

Certain scents activate smell receptors in the nose, which trigger a reaction in the nervous system, stimulate the part of your brain and trigger the release of feel-good neurotransmitters. Studies in the *International Journal of Molecular Sciences* have found that inhaling essential oils, like lavender, can lead to the release of serotonin and dopamine, key neurotransmitters associated with feelings of well-being and stress relief (Fung et al., 2021).

For instance, vanilla is known for its antidepressant and pain-reducing effects, lavender to induce calm and sleep, eucalyptus for seasonal allergies and cleansing the respiratory system of excess mucous and so on.

Does this mean that using essential oils alone will drive away all your stress? No, you must address the root cause and work on your mindset, beliefs and perspective.

How to Use Calming Scents

- Pick the right quality of essential oils known for their calming properties, such as lavender, chamomile, eucalyptus, vanilla or sandalwood.
- Add a few drops of essential oils to water and use it with a diffuser. As it disperses, inhale deeply to feel an immediate calming effect.
- You can dilute the essential oil with a carrier oil like, coconut or almond oil, before applying it to pulse points like your wrists, temples and behind the ears. Try a patch test on the inside of your wrist first to rule out allergies.
- A gentle scalp or foot massage with lavender or sandalwood can help reduce stress and anxiety.
- Add a few drops of essential oil to your bathwater.
- You can also use natural-scented candles or incense sticks.
- To deepen your sleep quality, use an essential oil-infused pillow mist on your bedding before sleep.

- Use a blend of essential and carrier oils for a soothing self-massage.
- Practise mindful breathing while using aromatherapy. Close your eyes, take slow, deep breaths and focus on the scent.

Many cultures have embraced the calming power of scents through traditional practices.

- In Ayurveda, essential oils, such as sandalwood, rose and jasmine, are used to balance specific doshas (body-mind types). For instance, lavender is used to cool excess *pitta* (heat and fire), while sandalwood and rose support balance for *vata* (air and space).
- A centuries-old tradition in Japan uses different incense blends in ceremonies to elevate mood, increase focus and promote relaxation. *Kōdō* ceremonies involve burning specific wood types and herbs to bring a sense of balance and mindfulness.
- Persian and Middle Eastern *oud*, a resinous wood, has been burned and infused in oils for centuries to bring calmness and clarity. It is known for its grounding properties, often used in meditation and sacred spaces.

Experiment with scents that you find relaxing or comforting. Create your own aromatic sanctuary. Do this well.

57

Singing

Whether you are a charming, polished singer who can belt notes, or a bathroom singer, who prefers their talents to be hidden, we've got news for you. Singing is incredible to activate your PNS.

Let's test this out, shall we?

Try singing a line as you read this. Notice how it produces vibrations that resonate through your body, particularly your chest, throat and head? These vibrations have a calming effect, almost similar to the benefits of deep breathing exercises. Research in *Frontiers in Psychology* suggests that singing, especially when it produces certain frequencies, can stimulate your vagus nerve. It can also release dopamine, endorphins and serotonin, associated with pleasure, reward and feeling good (Vickhoff et al., 2013). According to a study in *Evolutionary Psychology,* this is why many people feel happier and less stressed after singing (Dunbar et al., 2012).

Try holding a note while you sing. Notice how it requires controlled breathing? This way, singing also encourages diaphragmatic breathing—a deep, slow breathing pattern that enhances oxygen flow and induces relaxation. According to the *American Journal of Respiratory and Critical Care Medicine,* group singing exercises can enhance lung function and reduce symptoms in patients with chronic obstructive pulmonary disease (COPD) (Marquis et al., 2020).

Did you know that your posture, while singing, also matters? Have you noticed how classical singers assume a straight posture, while sitting or standing, to sing? A proper posture supports efficient breathing and reduces tension in the body.

Singing is used as therapy in managing various health conditions. For instance, it is used in speech therapy for stroke patients, respiratory therapy for those with lung conditions and emotional therapy for mental health issues like depression and anxiety. Because it engages both your body and mind, it effectively reinforces muscle memory and cognitive function.

You may notice how among individuals with dementia, singing familiar songs can trigger memories and improve cognitive engagement. Even when verbal communication is impaired, musical memory often remains intact, allowing individuals to sing or recognize songs from their past.

Traditional Practices and Unique Traditions in Singing Therapy

Practised in India, *Nada Yoga* uses singing and chanting to enhance spiritual and physical well-being. Chanting sacred syllables, like 'Om', creates vibrations believed to calm the mind and align the body's energy. It's thought to be particularly beneficial for reducing stress and anxiety.

Many cultures use group singing for spiritual and emotional healing. Gospel choirs, popular in African-American communities, create a sense of unity and joy. The communal aspect of singing promotes social connection and mental resilience.

In Nordic traditions, *Kulning* is a unique vocal technique used by herders to call livestock across large distances. This traditional singing style has a strong, open resonance that stimulates the vocal chords and produces a soothing effect on both the singer and the listener.

Originating from Mongolia and Tuva, throat singing involves creating multiple pitches simultaneously. This technique produces vibrations throughout the body, which can stimulate the vagus nerve and help singers enter a relaxed, meditative state.

How Can You Embrace This Powerful Tool?

- Sing a favourite song or tune for a few minutes daily. Focus on each breath, the vibrations in your chest and throat and how your body feels. Try to observe the calming effect it has on your mind and body.
- Incorporate mindful singing into daily routines. In a quiet space, try singing a low tone that resonates in your chest. Hold the note and feel the vibration in your chest, allowing it to calm you. This exercise can be especially useful for releasing tension and grounding emotions.
- If you can't sing, try humming softly. This can still activate the vagus nerve and create a soothing vibration that helps you relax.
- Host group singing sessions, like a choir or karaoke night, in community centres, senior living facilities or even online. Pick a mix of familiar songs that evoke positive emotions and encourage everyone to participate, regardless of singing ability.

Singing is an uplifting, accessible and scientifically supported way to support your shift from SNS to PNS. Enjoy the experience and let the music take you to a state of peace and joy.

58

Sunlight

One of the most beautiful practices that I have been following myself and advocating to my clients, over the years, is waking up and soaking in your daily dose of sunshine.

There is an ease and warmth that embraces you when you close your eyes intently and immerse yourself completely in the magnificence of sunrises or sunsets. Over the years, thanks to the nature of my work, I have been able to enjoy the beauty of the most captivating and picturesque dawns and sundowns in different parts of the world.

It has become a tradition to enjoy the first and last sunrise and sunset each year. Many of my choicest memories have been around these sacred hours.

Why Sunshine Matters for Your Health

Why do I prescribe sunshine to people? Sunshine is a free medicine with which we are all blessed in abundance. It is a source of energy, happiness, life, sleep, mood and more. The sun is the giver of all life on earth—humans, animals, plants and other living beings.

Just 10 minutes of morning sunlight exposure can reset our circadian rhythms, promote restful sleep, enhance our digestive system, fortify our immunity, aid in muscle recovery and quality and even improve our eyesight. The sunlight hitting your eyes early in the day tells your body that it's time to wake up, while exposure to evening light helps wind down your system for rest. A study in *Sleep Medicine Reviews* found that exposure to morning light improves both the timing and quality of sleep by setting a healthy circadian rhythm (Cyr et al., 2022).

The sun's infrared rays, especially in the morning, act as potent antioxidants. These rays support immune health, improve muscle quality and recovery and relieve joint aches. Research published in the *Journal of Photochemistry and Photobiology B: Biology* shows that infrared light reduces inflammation and oxidative stress, aiding muscle repair and immune resilience (Yang et al., 2021).

You may have heard of the phrase, 'being a ray of sunshine in the dark', or someone lovingly asking a person, 'Aren't you a ray of sunshine?'

There is truth to it. Spending time in the sun can help activate the PNS, reduce stress and promote relaxation. This effect is partly due to the warmth of the sun, which can be soothing. Sunshine boosts the release of serotonin. This process explains the natural lift in mood that many people feel after spending time in the sun.

Sunlight is essential for Vitamin D synthesis. Beyond bone health and immune function, low Vitamin D is also linked to mood regulation and disorders. Studies in *Risk Management and Healthcare Policy* support this (Wang et al., 2023). This is why people going through emotionally turbulent times or illnesses are often recommended to go outdoors and soak in sunshine in their routine.

Have you heard of Seasonal Affective Disorder (SAD)? It is a type of depression that occurs at certain times of the year, usually in the winter, when daylight hours are shorter. The lack of sunlight can lead to decreased serotonin levels, contributing to symptoms of depression, lethargy and changes in sleep and appetite. If you live in a cold country with limited sunlight, this can be a big challenge. In these cases, exposure to the sun or even SAD lamps or light boxes that mimic natural sunlight may help, under the guidance of your expert.

Traditional Practices of Sun Exposure

You may have heard of *Surya Namaskar*, or Sun Salutations, but have you heard about sun gazing? It is an ancient practice, often done at sunrise or sunset, where gentle sunlight is believed to activate pineal gland functions, enhancing mental clarity and mood.

In Japan, the practice of forest bathing emphasizes the healing power of nature, including sunlight. Spending time in nature has been shown to lower blood pressure, improve mood and reduce stress. Japanese forest bathing incorporates early morning sun exposure to maximize these benefits.

Native American tribes incorporate sun rituals to connect with nature, focusing on the sun's warmth to support emotional well-being and physical vitality.

Embracing the Power of the Sun in Your Routine

- Aim for approximately 10–30 minutes of unprotected sunlight exposure, depending on your skin type, time of year and geographic location.
- It's best to seek gentle sunlight early in the morning or late noon or evening hours when UV rays are less intense.
- Start with short sessions, particularly if your skin is sensitive, and work your way up to 20 minutes. If you live in an area with high UV levels, adjust exposure times to minimize risk.
- Avoid peak sunlight when it can be harsh and cause sunburn. Consult a healthcare professional or dermatologist for personalized guidance on what and when the most suitable time for you is.
- Practise meditation, yoga or even mindful walking under sunlight to combine the benefits of sunlight with relaxation techniques. This helps boost serotonin and lowers stress.

- Embrace the habit of observing sunrises or sunsets as a family or personal tradition. These moments encourage gratitude and connection with nature, promoting emotional well-being.

The next time you see the sun, take a moment to let it warm your face, close your eyes and breathe deeply. Appreciate the simple, yet profound, benefits of sunlight, and allow it to enhance your health and well-being naturally.

59
Breath Counting

You may have heard about counting sheep when you struggle to fall asleep, but have you heard of breath counting? Known as *ganana* or *susoku-kan* in Zen Buddhism, it focuses on drawing attention to your breath by counting each round of inhalation-exhalation.

Breath counting has been a cornerstone of Zen meditation for centuries. It is believed to have originated in ancient Japan as a method to help monks develop concentration and mindfulness.

The simplicity of the practice makes it accessible to anyone, regardless of meditation experience, allowing individuals to harness the power of their breath to anchor their awareness in the present moment.

It can help you by:

- Focusing the mind and directing attention to the breath, gently guiding it away from distractions and intrusive thoughts, allowing a state of calmness and clarity.
- Activating the PNS with deep, rhythmic breathing patterns. Research published in *Frontiers in Human Neuroscience* found that slow, rhythmic breathing directly influences the brain's stress response system (Zaccaro et al., 2018).

- Encouraging you to be present fully and become more attuned to your inner state and the sensations of your breath, which is grounding. Research from the *Mindfulness Journal* suggests that breath-focused practices can increase self-regulation and reduce impulsive reactions (Ge et al., 2025).
- Helping you cultivate response over reaction by providing a steady rhythm that soothes your mind and body.
- Enhancing attention by training the mind to stay focused on a single task. A study from *Consciousness and Cognition* found that practices like breath counting improve sustained attention, providing a stable anchor for the mind (Chu et al., 2023).

Steps for Breath Counting

- Sit or lie down in a comfortable position with your back straight. Let your hands rest on your lap or by your sides.
- Gently close your eyes to minimize external distractions and bring your attention inward.
- Take a few deep breaths. Gently inhale through your nose and exhale through your mouth, to settle into the practice.
- Bring awareness to your natural breath, noticing the sensation of the air entering and leaving your nostrils.
- On your next exhale, silently count 'one'. Continue to count each exhale up to 'ten'.
- After reaching ten, return to counting 'one' on the next exhale. If your mind wanders and you lose count, gently bring your attention back to the breath and start again from 'one'.
- Keep your focus gentle and relaxed. The goal is not to control your breath but to observe and count it.

In the Thai Forest Tradition, monks use breath counting to strengthen mindfulness, count each exhale and re-centre themselves whenever distractions arise.

Aim to practise breath counting for 5–10 minutes daily, gradually increasing the duration as you become more comfortable with the practice, discipline and consistency.

Embrace this ancient practice to cultivate a tranquil mind and a serene heart. Whether you are seeking to reduce stress, enhance mindfulness or simply find a moment of stillness, breath counting is a gentle, yet powerful, practice to guide you towards relaxation and inner harmony.

60

Create a Nature Sounds Playlist

In the embrace of nature's quiet, the heart finds its own healing. One of the most cherished experiences of my life that I keep returning to is embracing the raw and all-consuming power of the wild. Every couple of years, I return to Ishara, in the heart of the Masai Mara in Kenya, which has become my home away from home.

The rustling leaves in a forest, the soothing flow of a stream, the distant call of birds and the rhythmic crash of waves can have a profound impact on our emotions and our souls. These natural melodies can lower stress levels, reduce anxiety and promote relaxation, helping to restore balance to our minds and bodies.

Nature's sounds are more than just pleasant to the ear; they connect us to a timeless rhythm. They bring a sense of calmness and peace, grounding us in the present moment and offering a respite from the chaos of daily life.

In a study from the *Proceedings of the National Academy of Sciences,* researchers found that natural sounds could even enhance cognitive function and creativity, making them useful tools for focus and productivity (Buxton et al., 2021).

In the Japanese practice of *shinrin-yoku*, or forest bathing, people find the time to reconnect with themselves and embrace emotional wellness through immersion in nature. Does this mean hiking through the woods? No. It uses the practice of connecting with nature through our senses of sight, hearing, taste, smell and touch.

Research in Japan on *Environmental Health and Preventive Medicine* has shown that spending time in forests and listening to natural sounds can significantly reduce stress, lower blood pressure and improve overall mental health (Li, 2022).

Bernie Krause, a renowned musician, soundscape ecologist, naturalist and bio-acoustician, has spent a big chunk of his life recording and studying the sounds of natural environments and habitats from various parts of the world—both on land and underwater. His work reveals how natural soundscapes can profoundly affect human emotions and well-being.

Managing PTSD with Nature-Based Therapy

Studies from the *Journal of Clinical Psychology* indicate that nature therapy can be beneficial for veterans struggling with PTSD, especially those who find traditional treatments challenging (Bettmann et al., 2021). Nature-based therapy (NBT) has shown promising results, such as reduced symptoms of anxiety, depression and overall PTSD severity. Veterans, engaging in outdoor activities or therapeutic programmes in natural settings, report a greater sense of calmness, improved focus and enhanced social connections, which collectively contribute to mental well-being. A 2017 review in the *Journal of Public Mental Health* notes that NBT positively influences veterans' mental health (Poulsen, 2017). Multiple studies echo these benefits, underscoring improvements in quality of life, hope and even workplace reintegration for some.

How can you benefit from the sounds of nature? Cannot take a trip to the wilderness? No problem. You can do this at home, too.

- Compile a playlist of your favourite nature sounds. This can include sounds like the soothing crash of ocean waves, rainfall, the chirping of birds or ambient tracks. Personalize the playlist to suit your mood and needs, whether for relaxation, focus or sleep.

- Integrate nature sounds into your meditation practice. This can enhance the meditative experience by providing a soothing auditory anchor that helps you connect more deeply with the present moment.
- Write down how listening to nature sounds makes you feel each day. Journalling can enhance your awareness of subtle shifts in mood and help you track the benefits over time.
- Attend or create your own sound bath sessions, where you immerse yourself in therapeutic sounds, including gongs, singing bowls or chimes. Music therapy sessions can also be beneficial, where music can address emotional, cognitive and social needs.
- Set aside time for mindful listening. Sit comfortably, close your eyes and focus solely on the sounds of nature or music. This could even be by your window or a surrounding park. Pay attention to the different elements, such as melody, rhythm and harmony, and notice how they affect your emotions and body.
- Use your nature sounds or music playlist during daily activities like reading, cooking or during a relaxing bath. This can help create a soothing environment and make these activities more enjoyable.
- Play nature sounds or calming music before bedtime to create a peaceful sleep environment. This can help reduce insomnia and improve the quality of your sleep. Research in *Frontiers in Psychology* has shown that exposure to natural sounds can encourage restorative sleep by lowering heart rate and breathing patterns (Ratcliffe, 2021).

In certain Native American practices, the sounds of running water, wind and animals are revered as spiritual guides and incorporated into daily rituals.

Whether you use it for background ambiance or to focus during your daily activities, use the sound of nature well.

61

Limiting Alcohol

In moments of stress, heartache or disappointment, many people reach for a glass of wine or a cocktail, seeking solace in the numbing effects of alcohol. Whether it's after a tough day at work, following a breakup or dealing with the betrayal of a friend, the allure of alcohol can seem like an immediate remedy—a temporary escape from emotional turmoil. However, what often begins as a simple coping mechanism can quickly morph into a detrimental cycle that ultimately exacerbates the very issues it sought to alleviate.

The Temporary High and the Deeper Low

While alcohol can provide an initial feeling of relaxation and euphoria, this effect is fleeting. The high that many experience is typically followed by a pronounced dip in mood, leaving individuals feeling more vulnerable and worse than before. This phenomenon occurs because alcohol acts as a depressant, suppressing the central nervous system and dulling emotional pain, but only temporarily. The emotions that were suppressed during drinking don't disappear; instead, they often resurface, often more intensely than before. This leads to a cycle of dependence where the individual finds themselves increasingly reliant on alcohol to mask feelings they are not yet ready to confront.

Scientific research underscores the neurobiological impacts of alcohol on the body. The *Journal of Psychoneuroendocrinology* indicates that alcohol consumption can lead to an increase in cortisol levels—our body's primary stress hormone. Elevated cortisol can contribute to feelings of anxiety and depression, creating a vicious cycle where the very substance intended to relieve stress actually exacerbates it. Increased cortisol levels can dysregulate the nervous system, resulting in heightened reactivity to stressors, mood swings and a diminished capacity for emotional regulation.

The Heart of the Matter: Alcohol and Emotional Pain

No amount of alcohol, regardless of its quality or price, can effectively resolve matters of the heart. While enjoying a fine bottle of wine in a celebratory setting is a different experience entirely, using alcohol to escape emotional pain is a form of avoidance. It's essential to recognize that alcohol itself is not the enemy. Instead, the responsibility lies with the individual and the intention behind their consumption.

Enjoying alcohol responsibly—acknowledging its role in social settings without allowing it to dominate one's emotional state—is a healthy approach. Cultures around the world, such as the French, often exemplify this. For them, sipping wine is an experience to be savoured, a celebration of the moment rather than a means of escapism. They drink not to drown sorrows but to enhance joy, illustrating that intention matters profoundly in how we relate to alcohol.

The relationship between alcohol and the nervous system is intricate. Alcohol consumption can disrupt the balance of neurotransmitters, chemicals responsible for transmitting messages in the brain. Initially, alcohol may enhance the activity of GABA, a neurotransmitter that promotes relaxation. However, prolonged use disrupts this balance, leading to increased excitatory neurotransmitters like glutamate, which can heighten anxiety levels over time. This dual effect can leave individuals feeling both relaxed and anxious, resulting in a state of dysregulation.

Moreover, research published on NCBI highlights the connection between alcohol consumption and sleep disturbances, which further exacerbate the stress response. Poor sleep quality can amplify feelings of anxiety and depression, creating a feedback loop that can be challenging to break. Instead of achieving a sense of calmness, individuals may find themselves in a heightened state of distress, struggling to regain balance in their lives.

To transition from a dysregulated nervous system to a balanced state, it's crucial to limit alcohol intake and explore healthier coping mechanisms. Acknowledging one's emotions, rather than suppressing them, allows for healing and growth.

It's important to differentiate between enjoying alcohol responsibly and using it as a crutch for emotional pain. Seek support from friends, family or mental health professionals if you need to.

Remember, it's not about the beverage itself but the relationship we cultivate with it. If you choose to consume alcohol, do it with the right intention and in a responsible manner. What you push down deeper often comes back with a vengeance.

62

Deep Conversations

Have you ever had a conversation that left you feeling lighter, seen and deeply connected? The kind that makes you lose track of time as you dive into thoughts, dreams and truths with someone who just gets you? You almost feel like they are your kindred spirit in that moment. These aren't just ordinary exchanges—they are deep conversations that can transform your state of mind and even your body's nervous system.

Something magical happens when we engage in deep, meaningful conversations. The heart opens, defences drop and the PNS—our body's rest-and-digest mode—takes the lead. The PNS is where we can breathe deeply, feel safe and connect authentically with others and ourselves.

Deep conversations create a sacred space where we can be vulnerable, without the fear of judgement. They allow us to share our stories, our fears and our joys in a way that feels nourishing—when we talk about what matters, like our dreams, struggles or even the simple moments that make us feel alive. Conversations that flow effortlessly, that dive beneath the surface, act as a gentle reminder that we're not alone. It's like an unspoken permission slip to release the weight we've been carrying and relax into the present moment.

The Science Behind Deep Conversations

A study published in the journal *Psychoneuroendocrinology* found that social bonding, through meaningful conversations, could trigger the release of oxytocin, leading to reduced stress and anxiety levels (Olff et al., 2013). This hormone encourages feelings of trust, safety and connection, which are crucial for activating the PNS. It's no wonder that after a heartfelt chat, you often feel like a weight has been lifted off your shoulders—that's your body physically responding to this deep connection.

Additionally, research shows that when we engage in emotionally supportive communication, our bodies produce more serotonin and dopamine—neurotransmitters associated with happiness and relaxation. Have you ever had a conversation where you truly felt heard—like the other person genuinely saw you for who you are? That's exactly what this study published in the *Journal of Positive Psychology*, rooted in Buber's existential dialogical theory, explores. It shows that when we feel valued and deeply listened to in a conversation, it's more than just nice—it actually boosts our emotional well-being. These everyday moments of connection, where we feel understood and appreciated, can do wonders for our mental health by giving us a real sense of worth in our relationships. (Fernández et al., 2025).

Another fascinating study from the *Proceedings of the National Academy of Sciences* found that people who frequently engage in substantial conversations report higher levels of life satisfaction and emotional stability (Collins et al., 2022).

Tips to Make the Most of Deep Conversations:

- Deep conversations start with active listening. Put away distractions, maintain eye contact and show genuine interest. Being present sends signals of safety and trust, allowing you and the other person to relax.
- Vulnerability is a beautiful way to connect, but it's important to gauge comfort levels. Share your thoughts and feelings authentically, but also respect when the other person needs space.

- Instead of yes-or-no questions, try asking things like, 'How did that make you feel?' or 'What's been on your mind lately?' These types of open-ended questions encourage deeper exploration and connection.
- Practise empathy, not judgement. Deep conversations aren't about solving problems; they're about connecting. Listen with empathy, rather than trying to fix or judge.
- Acknowledge what the other person is saying, with kindness and empathy. Reflecting on what you've heard or validating their feelings can deepen the bond and help both of you feel seen and heard.
- Create a comfortable environment. Whether it's a quiet café, a cosy spot at home or a peaceful park bench, the setting matters. A calm and comforting environment can make a conversation feel more intimate and help both of you relax.
- Don't feel pressured to fill every pause. Sometimes, a quiet moment can be just as powerful as words, allowing thoughts and feelings to settle and the PNS to take hold.
- Deep conversations don't have to be a one-time event. Following up with a message or sharing a related thought, later on, can keep the connection strong.
- When you go out with your partner, family or a friend for a lunch date or coffee, make a rule that neither of you can have your phones on the table, not even face down. Give yourselves the gift of undivided attention.

Deep conversations are more than just an exchange of words—they're a profound way to reconnect with yourself and others, creating a space for calmness, understanding and healing. In a fast-paced world, taking the time to slow down and truly connect isn't just valuable; it's essential.

63

Following Your Passion

Following your passion is one of the most profound ways to feel connected to your spirit. It's not just about finding joy; it's about tuning into a deeper, more grounded state of being. When we engage in activities that light us up—whether it's photography, music, art or learning a new skill that brings joy helps regulate a dysregulated nervous system.

Scientific research shows that when we are immersed in something we love, the brain releases dopamine, the 'feel-good' neurotransmitter, which helps reduce stress and increase a sense of calmness. It also reduces the production of cortisol, the stress hormone. This helps the nervous system switch from the sympathetic mode to the parasympathetic mode.

Activities that absorb our attention induce a flow state—a term coined by psychologist Mihaly Csikszentmihalyi—where we lose track of time and become fully immersed in what we're doing. This state allows us to disengage from external stressors, down-regulate the nervous system and access a deep sense of fulfilment.

For some, their job is their passion, and that's a beautiful integration. But for those who don't have that privilege, finding time to pursue personal passions, outside of work, is vital for emotional and physical well-being. It's not just a hobby—it's what your soul and spirit crave. When we nourish this connection, we naturally feel more at ease, grounded and, ultimately, happier.

In the famous Blue Zones—regions where people live significantly longer lives, like Okinawa in Japan or Sardinia in Italy—one common thread is that people have a passion, something they love and are dedicated to. For many, it's gardening, which connects them to the earth, provides a sense of purpose and engages them in a peaceful, calming activity that aligns with their natural rhythms.

Dan Buettner, who has studied Blue Zones extensively, and with whom I have had the privilege of connecting through my podcast, found that having a sense of purpose—what the Okinawans call *Ikigai*—is a critical factor for longevity. This sense of purpose often stems from engaging in a passion, which keeps the mind active, the body moving and the spirit nourished.

Research from Harvard's Department of Psychology supports this, showing that individuals who regularly engage in passion-driven activities tend to have lower rates of stress, higher levels of happiness and a greater sense of overall life satisfaction. In fact, a study published in *Lancet* showed that individuals with a strong sense of purpose had a 15 per cent lower risk of early death compared to those who felt less fulfilled.

Beyond the scientific data, the act of following a passion is one of the most effective ways to feel grounded. When we engage in something we love, we are present. It pulls us away from our worries, our scattered thoughts and our to-do lists, allowing us to come back to ourselves. Passion connects us to the present moment, where true peace exists.

For anyone who doesn't have a passion built into their job, it's crucial to carve out time. Whether it's painting, playing an instrument or simply cooking a meal with love, these activities feed the spirit in ways that are hard to quantify but easy to feel. It's what the soul needs, and the more connected we are to that, the more at peace and fulfilled we become.

64

Movement and Exercise You Enjoy

Movement is primal to human beings. Evolutionally, our bodies were made to move. Yet modern life has forced us into a sedentary lifestyle, where sitting for hours is the norm. Science has been sounding the alarm on this.

A review in *Comprehensive Physiology* emphasized that regular physical activity is one of the most effective ways to combat the health risks associated with prolonged sitting (Booth et al., 2012). Movement, in any form, helps to counteract the negative effects of our desk-bound lives, bringing us back to what our bodies are designed to do.

Beyond its obvious physical benefits, even science has long recognized that movement is the key, not just to physical fitness, but also to mental well-being, offering a natural way to down-regulate our nervous system and return to a state of balance, calm and clarity.

When we move, our bodies release a symphony of chemicals that can shift our state of mind. Physical activity increases the production of neurotransmitters like dopamine and serotonin, the same chemicals that many antidepressant medications aim to boost.

A study published in *Sports Medicine* highlights that regular exercise improves mood and emotional resilience by enhancing these neurotransmitter levels (Meeusen and De Meirleir, 1995). The result? A more relaxed and happier you, ready to take on whatever comes your way.

If you've ever experienced the 'runner's high'—that euphoric feeling after a great run—you've encountered the magic of endorphins, the body's natural painkillers. This surge, often described as a feeling of lightness and joy, can make a tough day seem a lot more manageable. It's a natural, chemical reset for your nervous system.

Interestingly, exercise acts as a form of positive stress, also known as hormesis. When you challenge your muscles, heart and lungs, you introduce stress to your body. Instead of harming you, this stress prompts your body to adapt, grow stronger and become more resilient. A study in the *Journal of Applied Physiology* emphasizes that moderate exercise can improve the body's response to stress by enhancing resilience at the cellular level (Radak et al., 2008).

However, like anything, balance is key. Overtraining, where you push your body beyond its recovery limits, can spike cortisol levels—the stress hormone—leaving you feeling more anxious rather than less. Conversely, under-training can leave you feeling sluggish, without tapping into the powerful benefits that movement offers. The goal is to find a sweet spot, where exercise invigorates you without pushing you into burnout.

A well-rounded exercise plan is about more than just burning calories or building muscle. It's about nurturing all aspects of fitness to keep your body and mind in harmony.

Here's what a holistic exercise plan involves:

1. **Strength Training:** Building lean muscle is not just about aesthetics; it's about creating a foundation of strength that supports everyday activities and keeps your metabolism robust. Strength training stimulates muscles, encouraging the release of growth factors that support brain health (Cotman et al., 2007). This doesn't always mean hitting the gym. Bodyweight exercises like squats, lunges, push-ups and planks can be just as effective in building muscle and promoting stability. These exercises use your own

body as resistance, making them accessible and easy to do anywhere.

Grip strength is another often-overlooked component of strength training that can be a powerful indicator of overall health. Studies have shown that grip strength is associated with longevity and heart health, as it reflects the condition of your muscles and nervous system. Incorporating exercises like deadlifts, pull-ups, dead-hangs or even simple farmer's walks can help improve grip strength, which translates into better performance in both fitness and daily activities. One can also invest in a portable hand-gripping device and adjust the resistance to build grip strength.

By building the strength of our grip, we send a signal to the brain that we are capable and able-bodied, reinforcing a sense of vitality and resilience.

Lifting weights doesn't just build biceps—it lifts your mood too. There's a certain joy in feeling capable and strong, especially when you push past your perceived limits. Lifting weights stimulates the release of brain-derived neurotrophic factor (BDNF), a protein that supports brain function and resilience. Studies have shown that this release contributes to better cognitive function and a reduced risk of depression (Cotman and Berchtold, 2002). Think of it as a brain boost that comes from picking up those dumbbells! It's no wonder that many find a sense of empowerment when they see themselves lifting more, feeling stronger and standing taller.

2. **Cardiovascular Health:** Cardio workouts, like running, cycling or swimming, boost your heart health and improve your VO2 max—your body's ability to use oxygen efficiently. Studies published in the *Neuroscience & Biobehavioral Reviews* show that even moderate cardio exercise can significantly lower stress levels and improve heart rate variability,

a key marker of nervous system balance (Thayer et al., 2010).

3. **Endurance and Stamina:** Building endurance helps your body adapt to longer periods of activity, increasing your capacity to manage stress without feeling fatigued. This resilience translates into daily life, making you better equipped to handle both physical and mental challenges.
4. **Mobility and Flexibility:** Incorporating yoga or stretching not only prevents injuries but also enhances the mind-body connection. Slow, mindful movements promote relaxation and stimulate the PNS, known as the 'rest-and-digest' mode. A study in *Evidence-Based Complementary and Alternative Medicine* noted that regular yoga practice can decrease cortisol levels, aiding in stress management (Cohen et al., 2007).
5. **Balance:** As we age, maintaining balance becomes crucial for preventing falls and maintaining coordination. Practices like Tai Chi improve balance and enhance focus and relaxation. It's a gentle, yet powerful, way to keep the nervous system steady.

Movement Should Be Enjoyable, Not Forced

One of the most important lessons about exercise is that it should feel enjoyable, not like a chore. If you're dragging yourself through a workout that you loathe, you're missing the point—and potentially sabotaging the benefits.

Research published in the *International Journal of Behavioral Nutrition and Physical Activity* shows that people who enjoy their exercise are more consistent and experience greater mental health benefits than those who feel forced into activity (Teixeira et al., 2012).

The key is to find what lights you up, whether it's a walk in the park, a dance class or a game of tennis. Start small. Start with 5 minutes. Later on, build it to 10 minutes, then 15 minutes and so on. Remember, no 'ego lifting'—listening to your body and choosing activities you love are far more important than pushing yourself into discomfort just for the sake of it.

Exercise isn't just something you check off a to-do list; it's a chance to connect with your body, to feel alive and resilient. It is a privilege to exercise. You *get* to move, strengthen and care for your body—not because you have to, but because you have the ability to. This mindset can make all the difference, turning exercise into an act of self-respect and gratitude, rather than a burden to bear.

65

The Art of Connection

Let's be real. We all want to feel connected. We are social beings who crave connection and belonging. Whether it's with our family, friends, partners or even colleagues, the relationships we build give our lives their deepest meaning. In my own practice, I continue to learn many such lessons from my end-of-life patients. I learned the same from my Dad, a week before he died.

When someone is approaching death, they do not talk about who they were, their bank balance, the position they held, the accolades they won or how much success they garnered. They talk about love, relationships they treasured or lost, memories, funny stories, who they will miss and regrets about what they did or didn't do.

A week before my Dad passed on, as I was by his bedside, we spoke about death. I asked him, 'What are you scared of?' He said, 'Leaving all of you behind. I will miss you all.' Yes, he also said that he would miss his plants and trees because he was an avid gardener.

It taught me something. While we are all of different ages with different dreams and ambitions, we can learn to build and nurture what is truly important in life now and at the end. It's easy to get caught up in the rush of life and forget to nurture the relationships that matter.

You've probably heard this before, but the quality of our relationships has a huge effect on how we feel day to day. Science backs this up in ways you might not expect. Take the Harvard Study of Adult Development, for example. It's one of the longest-running studies on human happiness and well-being. After following people for over seventy-five years, researchers concluded that having strong, positive relationships is the biggest predictor of a happy and healthy life—more so than career success, fame or even money. It's a powerful reminder of how much relationships shape who we are and how we experience life (Hart, 2023).

What Does Science Say About This?

People with strong social ties are less likely to suffer from mental health issues like depression or anxiety. One study published in *PLOS Medicine* found that those with solid social relationships had a 50 per cent better chance of survival than those without. It's not just about living longer but living better (Holt-Lunstad, Smith, and Layton, 2010).

Research by Sheldon Cohen at Carnegie Mellon University shows that people who feel supported by their loved ones experience less stress (Cohen and Wills, 1985). Less stress means fewer physical problems down the road, like heart disease, and even a longer life.

Here's a fascinating one: having close connections can make your immune system stronger. A study published in *Psychological Science* found that people with more social ties were less likely to get sick when exposed to cold viruses. It turns out that love and friendship might just be better than chicken soup for the immune system (Cohen et al., 2003).

As we get older, being socially connected can protect our cognitive abilities. A review in *Ageing Research Reviews* found that seniors who stay socially intergenerationally engaged have a lower risk of cognitive decline (Krzeczkowska et al., 2021). So, nurturing relationships could be a way to keep your mind sharp as you age.

Science makes it clear: the relationships we nurture have tangible benefits.

How to Build and Maintain Positive Relationships

- **Be a Good Listener:** It sounds simple, but actively listening to someone—listening, without distractions—can transform your relationships. People feel valued when you give them your full attention. The next time you're having a conversation, put down the phone, focus on what the other person is saying and ask questions that show you're engaged. You'll be surprised at how much closer this can bring you to others.
- **Show Appreciation Regularly:** Don't wait for a special occasion to show someone you care. Whether it's a quick text to say 'thank you' or a heartfelt compliment, expressing gratitude strengthens emotional bonds. Studies show that practising gratitude in relationships can lead to greater satisfaction and connection.
- **Practise Empathy:** Empathy is about putting yourself in someone else's shoes. When someone shares their feelings or experiences with you, try to understand where they're coming from, even if you don't fully relate. Empathy builds bridges, especially during conflicts or tough times, and makes others feel truly heard.
- **Make Time for Relationships:** Life gets busy, but one of the most important things you can do is prioritize time with people who matter. It doesn't have to be a grand gesture—even a simple phone call or meeting up for coffee can keep a relationship thriving.
- **Handle Conflict with Care:** Disagreements happen, but how we approach them can either strengthen or weaken our relationships. Instead of blaming or getting defensive, try to approach conflict with understanding and a willingness to find a solution.

> Sometimes, simply acknowledging the other person's feelings can de-escalate a situation.

At the end of the day, we all crave meaningful connections. Maybe it's time to reach out to an old friend, invest more time in a current relationship or start building new connections.

Whatever you choose, remember that nurturing positive relationships is one of the best investments you can make for your own happiness and health. The next step is simple: be intentional, present and open. You'll be amazed at how your life transforms when you make genuine connections a priority.

66

Appreciation for Self and Others

When I consult with my patients, I love to talk about their lives—especially moments that made them happy or feel accomplished. The instant switch I see in them during these conversations is amazing. These stories inspire and help them tap into their inner strength on their journey to managing their disease and recovery. I've noticed how delighted they are when given the chance to share something they're proud of. It's like watching a child light up when they tell you about their achievements with the widest smiles. What are they looking for? To share their joy and get appreciation. The truth is that every human being wants to feel acknowledged and validated, but in the right way. We need to be mindful and aware when someone is sharing an accomplishment or story with us. Take the time to ask them more about it and genuinely appreciate them.

Appreciation, or gratitude, is not just a feel-good concept; it's a scientifically supported practice with measurable benefits for both the giver and the receiver.

According to research published in the *Journal of Personality and Social Psychology*, individuals who expressed gratitude or appreciation to their partner felt more positively about the relationship and were more committed to making it work (Gordon et al., 2012). Similarly, receiving appreciation from others makes people feel valued, leading to closer and more trusting bonds.

Studies in *Personality and Individual Differences* show that people who regularly practise appreciation report fewer physical symptoms, such as headaches or fatigue, and even experience better sleep quality (Hill, Allemand, and Roberts, 2013).

How Do You Tap into Appreciation for Yourself and Others?

Most of us find it easier to show appreciation for others than for ourselves.

Self-appreciation, however, is just as important. It's about recognizing your own worth, celebrating your accomplishments and being kind to yourself, especially during difficult moments.

Here are some simple ways to do that:

- **Take time each day to reflect on what you did well.** This doesn't have to be grand—maybe you handled a stressful situation with grace or took a step towards a personal goal. Celebrating these small victories fosters a positive relationship with yourself. Give yourself some credit when it is due. Write or record a note appreciating yourself. When you are feeling down, revisit these. Simply look in the mirror and acknowledge something you're proud of.
- **When things go wrong, or you make a mistake, it's easy to be critical. But try self-compassion, for a change.** It is about treating yourself with the same kindness you'd show a friend. Studies by psychologist Kristin Neff have shown that practising self-compassion leads to lower levels of anxiety and depression and boosts overall well-being (Neff, 2009).
- **Our bodies and minds work hard every day. Show appreciation by taking care of them**—whether through mindful movement, eating nourishing foods or simply resting when needed. As clichéd as it might

sound, your body is a temple. Expressing gratitude for your body can transform your relationship with it.

Showing appreciation for others can be as simple as saying 'thank you', but its effects are far-reaching. Here are a few ways to express it meaningfully:

- Instead of a general *'thank you'*, try to be specific about what you appreciate. For example, *'I really appreciate how you helped me with that project last week. It made a huge difference.'* Specificity not only makes your appreciation feel more genuine but also deepens the emotional connection.
- Surprise someone with an unexpected note or gesture of appreciation. This could be a handwritten letter, a small gift or even a thoughtful message.
- It's easy to appreciate someone for the big gestures, but don't overlook the small, everyday acts. Whether it's a partner who makes your coffee in the morning or a friend who listens when you need to vent, acknowledging these little moments can strengthen your relationship immensely.

How Emma Learnt to Appreciate Herself

I was consulted by Emma, a twenty-eight-year-old, during a particularly tough time in her life. Emma had always been the strong one in her family, the one everyone leaned on. But after her father passed away, suddenly, she found herself spiralling into grief and self-doubt. She started feeling disconnected, not just from the people around her, but from herself. Every day felt like a struggle, and the weight of her responsibilities seemed overwhelming. She began to wonder if she was even doing anything right.

One evening, as Emma was sorting through her father's belongings, she came across a small journal. Inside, she found pages filled with little notes of appreciation he had written for her over the years. *'Emma always knows how to make me smile, even on my worst days.' 'So proud of Emma for finishing her degree—she worked so hard.'* These notes weren't fancy, but they were heartfelt, and they reflected how deeply her father had valued and appreciated her.

Reading through those notes, Emma felt something shift within her. It was as though she could hear her father's voice, reminding her that she was enough—that she had always been enough, even during moments when she doubted herself. Slowly, she began to extend the same kindness towards herself. Each morning, we encouraged her to write down one thing she was proud of or grateful for in herself. Some days, it was as simple as *'I got through today'*, and on others, it was more profound, like *'I handled that difficult conversation with grace.'*

As her self-appreciation grew, she also began expressing more gratitude for the people in her life. She realized how much love and support she had, even in her darkest times. One day, she decided to write a letter to her brother, thanking him for his patience and understanding through her grief. That letter deepened the connection between them, and they began to talk more openly about their feelings.

I believe appreciation is not just about feeling good in the moment, but about creating a mindset that sees value in ourselves and the people we encounter. So, take a moment today to appreciate the small things—both in yourself and in others. Do this well.

67

Unplugging to Reconnect

You and I live in a hyper-connected world, where the constant buzz of notifications, endless news cycles and often toxic social circles can drain our emotional energy. I've noticed, in my own life, how liberating it is to simply step away from it all. To unplug, quieten the noise and reconnect with what truly matters. Last year, my team and I decided to go off social media for eight days, and the results each team member shared were simply spectacular.

The small act of disconnecting can bring immense relief and significantly improve emotional well-being by moving you from an always-alert mode to a state of relaxation.

Have you ever thought how easily time slips away while scrolling through videos or posts on social media? How it starts as that one video while you're waiting for a meeting to start. A few short videos later, you realize 30 minutes have passed! And you cannot even recall what you watched first! This isn't just mindless scrolling. It's a dopamine-driven cycle that affects our brain health and mental clarity.

We live in an age where information flows non-stop, and our gadgets are a gateway to the world. Yes, technology is excellent, but it can also overwhelm us.

The 24-hour news cycle bombards us with stories of crisis, disaster, war, violence and conflict. Social media, on the other hand, through rose-tinted glasses and filters, pulls us into a comparison trap, leaving many of us feeling inadequate or anxious. While it seems like staying plugged in is the only way to keep up, research shows that stepping back can be far more beneficial for our mental health.

The Science Behind Disconnecting

There is growing research supporting the idea that disconnecting from negativity—whether it's news, social media or unhealthy relationships—has tangible benefits.

- A study by the *British Psychological Society* found that participants who consumed constant negative news reported being more anxious and less hopeful about their own lives (de Hoog and Verboon, 2020). Disconnecting, even temporarily, helps lower those stress levels.
- *The National Sleep Foundation* (2022) reports that people who are glued to their devices before bedtime often experience poorer sleep quality, leading to fatigue and irritability the next day. Disconnecting from screens can not only reduce the emission of blue light that suppresses melatonin, your sleep hormone, but also helps with emotional stability.
- Constant multitasking—flipping between apps, emails and social media—makes it hard to focus. Research from Stanford University shows that multitasking can reduce productivity and increase mental fatigue (Madore et al., 2020). When we disconnect from our devices, we're able to focus more on the present moment, which reduces feelings of being overwhelmed and helps us feel more grounded.
- Surrounding yourself with negativity—whether through toxic relationships, unhealthy social circles or constant exposure to the misfortunes of others—drains emotional energy. A study in the *Journal of Personality and Social Psychology* found that people who regularly disengage from negative relationships

report improved mood, higher self-esteem and greater emotional resilience (Harris and Orth, 2020).

Let me give you an example from our life coaching sessions. A teenager came to us, overwhelmed by anxiety and crippling self-doubt. When we got down to addressing the root cause, we realized she was consumed by the constant need for validation from social media, where she compared herself to unrealistic standards. It became clear that her emotional health was deteriorating under the weight of this digital pressure.

We worked together to understand the toll social media was taking and introduced the idea of slowly disconnecting. At first, it was hard for her to let go—her phone had become a lifeline to a world of curated perfection. But we encouraged her to experiment with small steps: setting boundaries around her screen time, unfollowing accounts that made her feel inadequate and focusing on what truly brought her joy offline.

As she began to disconnect from social media, she reconnected with herself. Instead of mindless scrolling, she filled her time with art and journalling, activities that allowed her to express her authentic self. The transformation was remarkable. Within weeks, her anxiety lessened, and she began to feel more confident in who she was—outside of the digital lens. She no longer sought approval through likes or comments, and her sense of worth grew from within.

By disconnecting, she found emotional freedom. It wasn't just about putting down the phone but reclaiming her sense of identity and self-worth.

Some Practical Tips for Disconnecting

- **Instead of constantly scrolling through news feeds, designate a specific time to catch up on important headlines.** Consider opting for news summaries that keep you informed without overwhelming you.
- **If certain accounts make you feel anxious, envious or drained, unfollow them.** Curate your social media

feeds to include uplifting, positive content that adds value to your life.

- **Set aside time each day or week to disconnect from your devices completely.** Spend that time engaging in activities that bring you joy—reading, exercising or simply enjoying quiet time with loved ones.
- **Turn off notifications from unimportant apps, or uninstall the ones that do not add value.** Delete apps that you know are a mere distraction, which you can do without.
- **Plan your social media time into your daily schedule,** and only check emails and other trivial browsing in the time that you have allotted for it. It is crucial to access social media with an intention. Because, without it, we are bound to end up scrolling mindlessly.
- **Try taking a walk without your phone and notice how much more present and alive you feel.** You can even decide to leave the phone behind when you step out for your walk or your grocery shopping and so on. This will enable you to observe the world around you. You might notice things that you otherwise would not while you walk around looking down at your phone's screen. Rather than having your earphones on, listen to the sounds around you. You will be surprised by the different kinds of sounds you come across when you listen deeply. It is also a very meditative experience to soak in surrounding sounds mindfully.
- **Take a step back from people who drain your emotional energy.** It's important to surround yourself with supportive and positive influences.

Remember, disconnecting isn't about shutting the world out; it's about tuning into what truly matters. Take a moment to unplug, look up and focus on the present. You might be surprised at how much lighter and emotionally better you feel.

68

Cultivating Mindfulness

One lifestyle prescription I give most of my clients is getting started on **Vitamin M.** A few doses every single day. Wondering what Vitamin M is? It stands for **mindfulness**. I have experienced the benefits of this underrated practice in my own life.

The Oxford Dictionary defines mindfulness as the quality or state of being conscious or aware of something. Allow me to contextualize it for you. Mindfulness is a superpower you already possess. All you need to learn is to pause, take a step back and channel it.

Does mindfulness mean isolating yourself in a room and chanting affirmations or meditating for hours? No. It simply refers to a state where you focus on the present and become fully aware of where you are and what you are doing.

You can practise it anywhere and at any time—while you are tying your shoelaces, taking a shower, working, listening to music, taking a walk or even waiting in a queue!

The Science of Mindfulness

- Research by Harvard Medical School shows that mindfulness reduces the size of the amygdala, the brain's fear centre, helping with stress and anxiety (Hölzel et al., 2013).
- Another study in *Psychiatry Research* found that mindfulness increases grey matter in the brain,

enhancing empathy, memory and learning (Hölzel et al., 2011). It doesn't just calm the mind; it rewires it for resilience.

Only when we emulate the goodness of this practice in our daily lives do we learn to make the right decisions for our health. When we are mindful, we choose to eat better, sleep better, work out, meditate and rest when our bodies need a break.

Remember, we can follow the best nutritional plans or programmes. However, mindfulness is that special ingredient that allows us to grow and bloom in all aspects of human life, right from our health, relationships, personal growth, business, career and so much more.

Can mindfulness transform the way you are living? Yes, it absolutely can. My team and I have led close to 3,000+ participants on mindfulness journeys over the years. Thanks to the thousands of people we have coached through this mindfulness journey, we can confirm that the key to bridging the gap between motivation and action is **Vitamin M.**

Living with awareness in everything you do, no matter how small or big the task is, can be a game-changer in helping you achieve your goals.

Most of us talk, read about and try to practise mindfulness. But the truth is that very few of us really put in the effort to apply it to our daily lives. For instance, we practise our breathing techniques diligently during morning yoga. However, how many of us allow the essence of yoga to slip effortlessly into the rest of the day?

Let me ask you. How many of you remember the taste of the sip of tea you took yesterday or the meal you ate? Do you remember how that last hug from your loved one felt? No, right?

It is because we are moving very fast. In the process, we miss out on the little things that have the greatest impact. Without mindfulness, we are just reacting to everything around us—people, events, work and emotions. The resulting stress from these is the root cause of every single disease. With mindfulness, we train our minds to focus on and appreciate the things around us.

From listening to the sounds around you, focusing your breath, walking barefoot, feeling the cool breeze or even having a good cry—it could manifest itself in different ways. Any mundane activity can be done mindfully. You only need to add a pinch of mindfulness to mindless actions.

It needs time, practice, dedication, self-restraint, an open mind and above all, trust in the process.

Simple Mindfulness Exercises

Savouring Small Moments

Choose a single daily activity (like drinking coffee) and focus on it completely. Notice every step, smell, taste and sensation involved, savouring the experience fully.

Mindful Posture Check

Pause a few times throughout the day to check your posture. Bring awareness to your alignment, breathing and any tension you may be holding.

Emotional Weather Report

Check-in with yourself and identify your emotional 'weather' (e.g., sunny, cloudy, stormy). Notice your emotions without judgement, letting them pass like weather patterns.

Finger Tracing Breathing

Trace one hand with the finger of your other hand. Breathe in as you trace up a finger, and breathe out as you trace down. Repeat for all fingers, focusing on your breath and touch.

Mindful Imagery

Close your eyes and picture a peaceful scene (e.g., a beach, a forest, a mountain). Imagine yourself there, immersing all your senses to experience the place fully.

Mindful Texting or Typing

Before sending any message or email, pause, take a breath and read over it mindfully. Notice the tone and intention behind your words.

Object Exploration

Hold an everyday object (e.g., a pen, a key, a leaf) and focus on it entirely for a few minutes. Notice its texture, weight, temperature and how light interacts with it.

Heartbeat Awareness

Sit quietly and try to feel your heartbeat without touching your chest or wrist. This exercise builds inner awareness and connection with your body's rhythm.

In my years of consulting, I've seen that people who adopt mindfulness into their daily routines—whether they're managing a disease or simply seeking greater well-being—experience more peace, better decision-making and greater self-awareness. Try one of these exercises today.

69

Finding Moments of Joy and Laughter Daily

When was the last time you laughed so hard that your ribs ached? Have you ever noticed how effortlessly babies or young children laugh? Their laughter is unrestrained, full-bodied and contagious. In the rush of our busy lives, it's easy to overlook these simple moments of joy. Yet, laughter is one of the most powerful medicines we have—it not only lifts our spirits and strengthens our relationships, but it also has profound benefits for our physical health, improving everything—from heart health to stress relief.

The Science Behind Laughter: Why It's So Powerful

Laughter is more than just a fleeting moment of joy—it triggers incredible changes in the body. What makes laughter so special is its effect on the brain. When we laugh, the brain releases dopamine, a neurotransmitter that contributes to feelings of pleasure and satisfaction. This makes us feel more optimistic and, over time, we become more resilient to stress.

- Studies published in *Current Research in Physiology* have shown that laughter reduces stress hormones, like cortisol and adrenaline, while also boosting feel-good endorphins (Akimbekov and Razzaque, 2021).

- A study published in *Scientific Reports* found that participants who watched a funny movie had significantly lower stress levels and improved immune function (Froehlich et al., 2021). Laughter has even been shown to lower blood pressure and improve cardiovascular health.
- Beyond the individual benefits, laughter also strengthens social bonds. According to research from the *Journal of Neuroscience*, laughing with others releases endorphins, which enhance feelings of connection and trust (Manninen et al., 2017). It's no wonder that sharing a good laugh can deepen friendships and ease conflicts. When we laugh together, we create positive memories and reinforce the bonds that keep us emotionally connected.

Laughter as Medicine: Healing Through Humour

There's a reason why the old saying, 'laughter is the best medicine', still holds true. Laughter therapy is used in hospitals across the world to aid in healing.

For instance, Hunter 'Patch' Adams, famous as Patch Adams, is an American physician, social activist and clown, known for pioneering the use of humour and compassion in healthcare. Born in 1945, Adams was deeply affected by the loss of his father and later, his own battles with depression. After recovering, he committed his life to making the world a more compassionate place. He founded the Gesundheit! Institute in 1971, which focused on patient care through laughter, friendship and kindness. His work even inspired the 1998 Robin Williams starrer, *Patch Adams*.

It is scientifically proven that laughter positively affects the neuroendocrine and immune systems. Let's break this down.

- The neurological system controls how we experience pain, pleasure and emotions. Laughter releases endorphins, which not only reduce pain but increase feelings of pleasure. A study published in *Proceedings of Biological Sciences* showed that participants who engaged in laughter saw a 25 per cent boost in pain tolerance (Dunbar et al., 2012).

- Laughter regulates hormones, helping manage metabolism, thyroid function and even autoimmune conditions. For people with diabetes, laughter can lower postprandial (after-meal) blood glucose levels. It reduces the growth hormone factor involved in conditions like arthritis and other autoimmune diseases, bringing the immune system into a calmer state.
- Laughter strengthens the body's defence mechanisms by boosting natural killer cells, which are responsible for identifying and eliminating viruses and cancer cells. The release of these cells enhances the body's ability to fight off infections and potentially reduces tumour growth.

The benefits of laughter go beyond short-term relief. Its impact on gene expression (how genes are turned on or off) shows that our environment, including emotions, like joy, can regulate genes related to conditions like diabetes, cancer and cardiovascular health.

How Laughter Heals: The Mind-Body Connection

The reason why laughter has such a profound effect on health lies in its ability to move us from the SNS to the PNS. This shift promotes relaxation, signalling to the body that it's safe and can heal.

When we laugh, our body naturally releases endorphins, reducing pain and creating a sense of euphoria. It also stimulates oxytocin, the 'love hormone', which strengthens bonds between people, making laughter a powerful social tool. In groups, shared laughter creates a sense of belonging, safety and connection.

Laughter is also effective in managing anxiety and depression.

Fun fact: Even forced laughter tricks the brain into releasing dopamine, the feel-good chemical, which improves mood and reduces feelings of stress. So, even when we don't feel like it, simply smiling or laughing can shift us into a better emotional state.

Laughter and Disease Management

- A study published in *Diabetes Care* found that laughter after meals significantly reduced postprandial blood glucose levels in Type 2 diabetes patients, suggesting laughter as an effective management tool (Hayashi et al., 2003).
- Laughter lowers the overproduction of growth hormones and calms the immune system to prevent it from attacking healthy tissues. Research in *Rheumatology* revealed that laughter therapy reduced inflammatory markers in patients with rheumatoid arthritis, calming the immune response (Matsuzaki et al., 2006).
- Research from the University of Maryland Medical Center (2025) shows that laughter relaxes blood vessels, improving circulation and reducing the risk of heart attacks and strokes.
- Laughter stimulates abdominal muscles, aiding in digestion by promoting the release of digestive enzymes and insulin from the pancreas.
- Research in the *European Journal of Pain* demonstrated that laughter triggered endorphin release, significantly increasing pain tolerance (Pérez-Aranda et al., 2019).

The Importance of Finding Daily Joy

Incorporating laughter into our daily lives isn't just about entertainment—it's about finding balance amidst life's challenges.

I've personally seen how laughter changes lives. One such remarkable story involves a fifty-three-year-old woman named Maya, a cancer patient I worked with. Maya was initially resistant to the idea of finding joy in such a dark time, but as part of her treatment plan, we incorporated laughter therapy. She started watching her favourite comedies and invited friends over for light-hearted game nights. In those moments of laughter, Maya found a sense of freedom from her pain and fear. She felt more hopeful, and her doctors noted how her mood and energy levels improved.

How You Can Cultivate Laughter Daily

Finding moments of joy and laughter doesn't have to be complicated. Here are some ways to bring more laughter into your life:

1. **Watch or Read Something Funny:** Whether it's a comedy show, a funny YouTube video or a humorous book, make time for content that makes you laugh. Just 15 minutes a day can significantly improve your mood and health.
2. **Spend Time with Funny Friends:** Surround yourself with people who bring out the best in you. Laughter is contagious, and being around joyful people can lift your spirits.
3. **Laugh at Yourself:** Learn to see humour in your own mistakes. Taking yourself less seriously allows for a more relaxed, joyful approach to life.
4. **Create a Laughter List:** Recall memories that make you laugh, to turn to when you're stressed.

Laughter may not solve every problem, but it gives us the strength to face them. When we seek out joy and laughter, we transform our mood, our relationships and our overall health. I invite you to make space for laughter in your life. Even in difficult times, moments of joy are always waiting to be found. Take a moment each day to seek something that makes you laugh—it might just be the medicine you need.

Laughter is not a replacement for medicine, but it is a powerful addition. It's a part of what I call 'medicine beyond medicine'—like sunlight, fresh air, good food and rest. These things don't replace treatments like chemotherapy or medication, but they significantly enhance the body's ability to heal. Embrace this simple gift that we all have access to—laugh more, love more and live more.

70
Crying

Crying often gets a bad rap because it's associated with sadness or vulnerability. But you know what? It may be good for you.

Think about this. When a baby enters the world, what is the first sign the doctors look for? The cry. When someone goes through a traumatic event or experiences grief, what is the natural reaction that is necessary for their body to go through? Tears.

When you cry, especially those good, soul-cleansing tears, it's like hitting a reset button for your emotions.

Crying is a natural way for your body to release pent-up emotions. When you let those tears flow, it's like letting go of all that emotional baggage weighing you down. It's like giving your mind a deep cleanse—it clears out the cobwebs and makes room for more positive thoughts and feelings.

But it's one of the most natural ways for our bodies to release tension, and it might even be essential for both our emotional and physical well-being.

Emotional Release: The Science of Letting Go

Studies show that emotional tears are chemically different from other types of tears, like reflex tears (which happen when something irritates your eyes). Emotional tears contain higher levels of stress hormones and toxins, including adrenocorticotropic hormone (ACTH), which plays a role in stress. According to Dr William Frey, a biochemist and expert on tears who authored *Crying: The Mystery of Tears* (1985), emotional tears release stress hormones, literally shedding stress as they fall.

The process of crying is part of the PNS's activation, a relaxation response in the body that helps us release tension and return to a calm state. A study from the *Frontiers in Psychology* journal notes that people often report feeling relief after crying due to this calming, restorative effect (Gračanin, Bylsma, and Vingerhoets, 2014).

Crying and Mood Regulation: Endorphins and Feel-Good Chemicals

One reason why you might feel lighter after crying is due to the release of endorphins. When you cry, your body releases oxytocin and endogenous opioids, often known as endorphins. These chemicals provide a numbing sensation that can ease both physical and emotional pain, leading to feelings of relief and calm. That's why after a good cry, you might feel strangely relieved and even a bit happier.

An article in the *Monitor of Psychology* points out that crying can lift your mood as these natural chemicals create a temporary sense of euphoria or well-being, similar to what we experience after exercise (Collier, 2022).

Tears as Natural Cleansers

Crying isn't just good for your mind—it can be good for your body too.

Tears serve as a defence mechanism, removing toxins from the body and cleansing the eyes of irritants. Reflex tears, which are produced when your eyes are exposed to something like smoke or dust, have been shown to contain antimicrobial proteins like lysozyme, which can kill 90–95 per cent of bacteria in a matter of minutes. Emotional tears also contain proteins and minerals that serve a cleansing function, flushing out impurities not only from the eyes but, metaphorically, from the mind as well.

Strength in Vulnerability: Crying as a Mark of Resilience

Research in *BMC Psychology* has found that those who are more in tune with their emotions, including crying, are often more adaptable and resilient to life's challenges (Zaid et al., 2025). Rather than suppressing emotions, releasing them through tears is a form of acceptance and self-compassion that can build our emotional strength.

Finding Comfort in Crying Traditions

Throughout history, many cultures have viewed crying as a powerful sign of inner strength. In Japan, *rui-katsu*, or tear-seeking events, encourage people to cry as a form of emotional release, believing it reduces stress and promotes group bonding.

In ancient Greece, public expressions of grief were seen as a sign of respect and humanity. Some indigenous cultures use crying as part of healing ceremonies, believing that tears connect them to the spirit world and help cleanse the soul.

In parts of Ireland, the traditional *keening* practice involves a mourning ritual that allows families and friends to cry openly as a sign of respect and healing. In some African cultures, communal crying is encouraged as a way to show solidarity and offer support to those in grief.

These practices reflect an understanding that crying isn't something to be ashamed of, but rather a natural, communal expression of emotion for healing.

Letting Go: The Next Time You Feel like Crying, Don't Hold Back

It's your body's sign that it needs a little tender loving care (TLC). Remember, crying isn't a sign of weakness—it's an act of self-care and a path to emotional resilience. Letting tears flow is a reminder of our humanity, a way to release the weight we carry and open the space for lighter, more positive feelings. Whether it's a tear-jerking movie, a painful memory or a burst of gratitude, allow yourself the release. Your mind and body will thank you for it.

71

The Power of Meditation

Meditation has been practised for thousands of years, not just as a spiritual practice but also as a tool for calming the mind and healing the body. It is one of the most important tools our integrative experts prescribe to our patients as a powerful bridge between the SNS and the PNS.

Ancient Techniques, Timeless Benefits

Ancient civilizations, from the yogis of India to the Zen masters of Japan, recognized the profound effects of meditation. These practices have stood the test of time, and modern science is now uncovering what ancient practitioners instinctively knew: **meditation calms the body, regulates stress and promotes healing.**

Scriptures from ancient traditions speak about the transformative power of meditation for the mind, body and soul. Across cultures, meditation has been viewed not only as a practice for spiritual enlightenment but also as a means to cultivate inner peace, self-awareness and connection to the divine. Let's dive into some of these, shall we?

What Do the Scriptures Say?

Vedas and Upanishads

In Hinduism, the Vedas and Upanishads, some of the oldest spiritual texts known to humanity, speak extensively about meditation, or *Dhyana*. The Upanishads describe meditation as a path to self-realization and unity with the universal consciousness, or *Brahman*. The scriptures emphasize that by quieting the mind and detaching from worldly distractions, one can experience *Atman* (the true self) and realize oneness with the divine. This idea is encapsulated in the phrase *Aham Brahmasmi*—I am Brahman.

In the Bhagavad Gita, Lord Krishna teaches Arjuna about meditative yoga, or Dhyana Yoga, as a way to achieve mental clarity and wisdom. Chapter 6 of the Gita focuses on how meditation can free the mind from fear, anger and attachment, leading one towards inner peace.

Buddhist Scriptures

Meditation is central to Buddhism, which emphasizes the practice of Vipassana (insight meditation) and *Samatha* (concentration meditation). The Pali Canon, a collection of scriptures in the Theravada Buddhist tradition, speaks about mindfulness (*Sati*) and right concentration (*Samadhi*) as key components of the Eightfold Path to enlightenment. Vipassana, for instance, encourages practitioners to observe their thoughts and bodily sensations without attachment, creating a deep awareness of impermanence and the nature of suffering.

The Buddha himself attained enlightenment through meditation under the Bodhi tree. His teachings, preserved in texts like the *Dhammapada*, guide practitioners to achieve liberation from suffering by calming the mind and cultivating mindfulness.

Christianity

While meditation may not be as explicitly mentioned as in Eastern traditions, the Bible alludes to contemplative practices. Psalm 46:10 says, 'Be still, and know that I am God.' Early Christian mystics, such as the Desert Fathers and St Teresa of Avila, practised a form of contemplative prayer that resembles meditation, known as *Lectio Divina*, where silence, scripture and mindfulness were used to draw closer to God.

Sufism

In the mystical Islamic tradition of Sufism, meditation is known as *Muraqaba*, a practice of focusing the mind on divine presence. The goal is to transcend the ego and experience *tawhid*, or the oneness of God. Sufi meditation often involves rhythmic breathing, repetition of divine names (known as *Dhikr*), and contemplation of the divine.

Ancient Forms of Meditation Practised Today

Many of the meditation techniques rooted in ancient traditions are still widely practised even today.

- Vipassana teaches you to develop a deep understanding of the transient nature of thoughts and emotions. Vipassana retreats, often lasting ten days, are held worldwide and continue to be a popular way for people to connect with this ancient technique.
- Derived from Vedic practices, Transcendental Meditation (TM) involves silently repeating a mantra for 15–20 minutes, twice a day. It is rooted in the ancient Vedic knowledge of mantras, which are believed to have vibrational qualities that calm the mind and elevate consciousness. It became popular in the twentieth century, and has gained millions of

followers, including celebrities and public figures, due to its simplicity and profound effects.

- Zen Meditation (*Zazen*), or seated meditation, involves sitting in a specific posture (often cross-legged), focusing on the breath and letting go of any attachment to thoughts that arise. The goal is to cultivate 'no-mind' *(Mushin)*, a state of total awareness, without judgement or attachment. Zen meditation is still widely practised in monasteries and by individuals around the world as a way to quieten the mind and experience deep insight.
- One of my favourite forms that I practise and encourage my clients to embrace is Metta Meditation (Loving-Kindness Meditation). It is where you cultivate love and compassion for yourself, loved ones, neutral individuals and even enemies. This ancient practice is still widely used today to help individuals develop empathy, reduce anger and foster emotional healing.
- Pranayama, mentioned in the Yoga Sutras of Patanjali, is a practice of controlling the breath to influence the flow of prana (life energy) in the body. Techniques like Anulom Vilom (alternate nostril breathing), *Kapalbhati* and *Bhastrika* are still widely practised today to calm the nervous system, improve mental clarity and promote overall well-being.
- *Qigong*, which translates to 'energy cultivation,' is an ancient Chinese meditation practice involving slow, meditative movements combined with breath control and visualization. This practice, used for both health and spiritual growth, is still popular worldwide, with many people practicing it to improve energy flow *(Qi)* and balance in the body.

The Science Behind Meditation: Moving from SNS to PNS

- Research has shown that just a few minutes of meditation daily can shift the body from a state of tension (SNS) to relaxation (PNS), enabling the body to repair, heal and maintain balance. A study in *Psychology Research and Behavior Management* shows mindfulness meditation as a self-help strategy to reduce anxiety and depression. It suggests that mindfulness can be a practical and effective tool for emotional regulation, especially when integrated into daily routines (Edenfield and Saeed, 2012).

- A Harvard Medical School study published in the *Journal of Brain and Cognition* showed that mindfulness meditation helps reduce the size of the amygdala, the brain's fear centre, thereby lowering stress levels and improving emotional regulation (Gotink et al., 2016).
- A 2011 study published in *Psychiatry Research* found that individuals who meditated regularly had increased grey matter in brain regions associated with emotional stability, memory and self-awareness (Hölzel et al., 2011).
- The *Journal of the American Medical Association (JAMA) Internal Medicine* published a meta-analysis in 2014 showing that mindfulness meditation programmes have moderate evidence of improving anxiety, depression and pain, making them an effective complement to traditional medical treatments (Goyal et al., 2014).

Integrating Meditation into Daily Life

When I first began meditating, I struggled too. However, early into my practice, I realized that meditation was not about forcing my mind to be still. It was about becoming aware of how thoughts came and went. How did I move from 5 minutes of meditation to 45 minutes? I was consistent with 5 minutes, then I added 2 minutes every alternate day. In less than 25 days, it happened. It's called the compounding effect and consistency with small wins.

During the first retreat I hosted in Ishara, Masai Mara, Kenya, some of my most cherished memories with our participants from various walks of life were the deep and reflective sessions and meditating in the wild.

You don't need hours in a cave or into the wildness or a perfectly quiet room to meditate. Even a few minutes of focused breathing can trigger the calming effects of the PNS.

Here are some simple, innovative ways to incorporate meditation into your daily routine:

- **Mindful Morning Routine:** Before you get out of bed, take a few deep breaths. Inhale for a count of four, hold for four and exhale for six. Focus on the breath and set an intention for your day.
- **Walking Meditation:** If sitting still feels daunting, try walking meditation. Focus on each step, feel the earth beneath you and synchronize your breath with your movements.
- **Mindful Eating:** Take a moment before eating to breathe deeply and express gratitude for your meal. Focus on each bite, the textures and the flavours. This not only promotes digestive health but also reduces overeating.
- **Breathing Breaks:** During the day, especially when you feel overwhelmed, take a 2-minute breathing break. Inhale slowly, hold for a moment and exhale deeply, relaxing your shoulders with each breath.
- **Progressive Relaxation:** This involves systematically tensing and then relaxing different muscle groups. It can be done sitting or lying down and helps release stored tension in the body. Before bed or upon waking, take 5 minutes to scan your body, mentally, from head to toe, focusing on each part with awareness.
- **Technology-Assisted Meditation:** Apps like Calm, Headspace and Insight Timer offer guided meditations ranging from 2 to 30 minutes, making it easy to practise anywhere.

- **Breathing as Meditation:** Whether in traffic, waiting in line or between meetings, take a few moments to focus on your breath. Even 2 minutes of deep, mindful breathing can reset your nervous system.
- **Meditation in Motion:** Explore practices like Tai Chi or Yoga, where movement and mindfulness intertwine, thus promoting physical and mental well-being.
- **Creative Visualization:** Incorporate visualization techniques into your meditation, imagining a peaceful setting, your goals or even a healing light surrounding you.

The beauty of meditation lies in its accessibility; it can be practised anywhere, at any time. Whether you have 5 minutes or an hour, this ancient practice has the potential to transform your health physically and mentally. Embrace the stillness, find your breath and allow meditation to guide you towards a more balanced existence.

72

The Science Behind Music

Music is a common thread that finds its place in most of our lives, no matter what the event. From daily walks to adventurous road trips, from birthdays to break-ups and marriages to funerals, it seamlessly fits into most aspects of our lives. Why?

Music is therapy for the human mind.

Close your eyes and think about the last time you heard a big group of people singing together. Was it a concert, a choir or a religious gathering? Remember the vibrations, energy and the goosebumps you felt with that collective singing? The harmonizing frequencies and rhythms, even if not perfectly matched, may have produced a pure vibration that made you feel good. A study in *Qualitative Health Research* has shown that group singing can elevate mood and reduce anxiety, making it one of the most powerful forms of community healing (Hendry, Lynam, and Lafarge, 2022).

Early in my career as a DJ, I experienced the power of music and the instant change of emotional energy it brought about in people. As an integrative practitioner, I continue to recommend it to this day.

For a long time, medical science has studied the effects of music on overall health, and the results have been nothing short of spectacular. Let's dive into the science behind this.

How Music Affects Your Brain

Music has a direct influence on the brain's neurochemical activity, particularly affecting serotonin and dopamine levels—the 'feel-good' neurotransmitters. When you listen to music you love, the brain releases these chemicals, improving mood and reducing stress.

Scientific research backs this up. A study from Stanford University showed that listening to rhythmic music could slow brainwave activity, helping to reduce anxiety and enhance focus. A Stanford University symposium titled *Brainwave Entrainment to External Rhythmic Stimuli* highlighted how rhythmic music can synchronize brainwaves—a phenomenon known as entrainment (2006). Slow rhythms may induce relaxed, meditative brain states, while faster rhythms enhance focus and alertness.

When we listen to or create music, the body shifts to the PNS, the body's 'rest-and-digest' mode. Music has been shown to reduce cortisol levels, lower heart rate and release endorphins, the body's natural painkillers and mood elevators.

A study published in the *Proceedings of the National Academy of Sciences* revealed that listening to music triggers the release of dopamine, the brain's pleasure chemical (Ferreri et al., 2019). Another study from *PLOS One* found that patients with anxiety and depression experienced reduced symptoms after regular music therapy sessions (Tang et al., 2020). By calming the nervous system, music therapy helps improve mental health, while promoting overall emotional balance.

How Music Helps Various Conditions

- **Anxiety and Depression:** Studies show that music significantly reduces anxiety levels by lowering cortisol and increasing serotonin. It may not solve every problem, but it makes coping easier. A study in the *Journal of Affective Disorders* revealed that music improved mood in depressed patients, making it a valuable tool for emotional healing (Marchetti et al., 2011; Gaebel et al., 2025). While it may not completely solve your problems, it can make you feel better.

- **PTSD:** Music can serve as a nonverbal form of therapy, helping those with PTSD manage stress. Its rhythmic and melodic patterns provide emotional release, often triggering calmness and reducing trauma-related symptoms.
- **Alzheimer's and Dementia:** Research in *Annals of the New York Academy of Sciences* has shown that Alzheimer's patients often recall memories associated with music from their youth (Matziorinis and Koelsch, 2022). A couple of years ago, a heart-warming video, showing a former ballerina with Alzheimer's, went viral as she gracefully danced in her wheelchair listening to Tchaikovsky's ballet *Swan Lake*. A study published in the *Journal of Clinical and Experimental Neuropsychology* found that patients exposed to familiar music had improved memory recall and cognitive function (Deason et al., 2019). Playing music from a patient's teenage years can spark emotional and cognitive healing, connecting them with forgotten memories. People with Alzheimer's respond best to music from their teenage or college years. It's amazing to see how these patients can connect this music to memories from that time.
- **Autism and Attention Deficit/Hyperactivity Disorder (ADHD):** Music therapy has shown great success in helping children with autism or ADHD reach developmental milestones. The rhythmic patterns of music help with attention span, motor coordination and communication skills.
- **Cancer:** Music is great for people who are going through cancer as well. We all know that cancer comes with its own fears. Music can help reduce your cortisol and adrenaline levels, and in turn, keep you calmer.

The calmer you are, the stronger your immunity, and the better your strength to manage your condition.

- **Blood Pressure:** Science is also showing us how music therapy can lower your blood pressure. So, if you suffer from high blood pressure, it can help you lower your blood pressure levels. It can help you lower inflammation in your heart, triglycerides and cholesterol levels. A study suggests that listening to Mozart for 25 minutes may lead to a reduction in blood pressure. The research, published in the journal *Deutsches Ärzteblatt International,* found that listening to music by Mozart and Strauss for 25 minutes had the effect of lowering both systolic and diastolic blood pressure (Trappe and Voit, 2016). Specifically, listening to Mozart or Strauss reduced systolic blood pressure by 4.7 mmHg and 3.7 mmHg, and diastolic blood pressure by 2.1 mmHg and 2.9 mmHg. Music by ABBA, however, had a smaller effect on blood pressure.
- **Chronic Pain and Surgery Recovery:** A systematic review and meta-analysis in the *Journal of Integrative and Complementary Medicine* shows that post-surgical patients, those who participated in music therapy reported significant reductions in pain compared to those who didn't (Li et al., 2024). The more we give something significance, the more it grows, whether it is with emotions or pain. If you're constantly thinking about your pains and aches, the more you feel it. Music serves as a distraction, reducing the brain's focus on pain, while also stimulating the release of endorphins—the body's natural painkillers.

The Simplicity of Music: Making It Work for You

You don't need formal training or music therapy sessions to benefit from music. Here are simple ways to add music to your daily life:

- **Create Playlists for Every Mood:** Design specific playlists for different moments—upbeat tracks for exercise, calming music like flute instrumentals for meditation, nostalgic songs to jog positive memories and soothing songs to peacefully end your day.
- **Play an Instrument:** If you know how to play, even casually strumming a guitar or tapping a drum can bring emotional release. Making music stimulates brain activity and enhances motor coordination.
- **Guided Meditation with Music:** Add instrumental music or Solfeggio frequencies to your meditation routine (read the next chapter in detail to know more).
- **Explore New Genres:** Don't limit yourself to one type of music. Experiment with classical, jazz and music from around the world. New rhythms and sounds stimulate brain activity and can lead to emotional growth. Challenge your brain by exploring unfamiliar music styles—jazz, classical or world music. Just because you grew up liking hip-hop, doesn't mean that you can't explore R&B, gentle, hard rock, psychedelic trance or classical music. Research published in *Brain, Behavior, and Immunity* shows that listening to new music can stimulate neurons and improve cognitive health (Zaatar et al., 2023).
- **Sing or Hum:** Singing, even alone, releases endorphins and reduces stress. If you're not comfortable singing, simply humming can have similar benefits by vibrating your vocal cords and calming the nervous system.
- **Try Instrumental Music:** If you're not into lyrical music, try instrumental music. Classical or ambient music, in particular, is known for its calming effects on the brain.

Music for Everyone

The power of music extends beyond clinical settings and reaches into our everyday lives. Beyond the psychological benefits, the actual vibrations from music affect the body's cells.

Every day, take a few minutes to explore the therapeutic effects of music. It could be as simple as taking 5 minutes, 10 minutes or 15 minutes, at intervals, to listen to your favourite music. You could start with one song, or maybe two. Just sit down, relax and listen to all your favourite songs. Sometimes, try it with your friends.

With scientific backing and countless real-life examples, the evidence is clear: music is beyond medicine—it is a natural healer, capable of transforming how we feel, think and heal. So, embrace its power today and every day.

73

Sound Therapy

Sound healing uses specific vibrations to calm the mind, ease tension and bring the body into balance. We incorporate this practice into our coaching, too.

A study published in the *British Journal of Health Psychology* found that listening to relaxing sounds led to significant decreases in cortisol levels, heart rate and blood pressure—showing how sound can help the body naturally shift from stress to relaxation (Chafin et al., 2004).

Some Types of Sound Healing Practices You Can Explore

- **Tibetan Singing Bowls:** Made of metal alloys, these bowls create deep, resonant sounds that are said to align chakras and bring emotional balance. Studies show that listening to Tibetan bowls can significantly reduce anxiety and depression symptoms. In fact, sound waves can physically affect the nervous system and organs. This is why Tibetan singing bowls, bells and chimes are often used in sound therapy, creating vibrations that ease tension and promote healing.
- **Crystal Singing Bowls:** These bowls, made from quartz, produce high-pitched tones believed to clear energy blockages. A study published in the *Journal of Evidence-Based Complementary and Alternative*

Medicine found that crystal and Tibetan bowls promoted deep relaxation and emotional healing in participants (Goldsby et al., 2017).

- **Gong Baths:** Gong baths involve immersing oneself in the sound waves of gongs. These vibrations penetrate the body and promote a meditative state. Research in the *Musicological Annual* shows that gong therapy can reduce stress and induce deep relaxation (Pesek and Bratina, 2016).
- **Tuning Forks:** Tuning forks are used to produce precise frequencies, helping to restore balance to the body's energy fields. Hold the vibrating fork near your body to release stress and restore harmony. Daniele Masala and Valentina Merolle authored an article titled 'The Tuning Fork and the "Soundtherapy"', published in *Senses and Sciences* in June 2017. This work explores the historical development and therapeutic applications of sound therapy, particularly focusing on the use of tuning forks. The authors discuss how specific sound frequencies can stimulate the body's energy systems, potentially aiding in self-healing processes. They highlight the contributions of pioneers like Sir Peter Guy Manners, who identified over six hundred healing frequencies corresponding to different body parts and emotional states. The article also examines Fabien Maman's integration of music and acupuncture, where tuning forks are applied to acupuncture points to harmonize the body's energy flow. The authors suggest that such sound therapy techniques may be beneficial in addressing various conditions, including chronic inflammation, arthritis and emotional imbalances.
- **Create Sound Healing Spaces and Rituals:** Set aside a room or corner in your home where you can play soothing music and relax. Play relaxing, healing sounds during your morning meditation or evening

wind-down routine to help regulate your nervous system and encourage emotional balance.

- **Solfeggio Frequencies:** These are a set of ancient musical frequencies, each thought to have unique healing properties—by far, one of my favourites that I have added to my own lifestyle and helped many patients embrace too. A study published in *Health* found that listening to certain Solfeggio frequencies (528 Hz) significantly reduced anxiety and improved mood (Akimoto et al., 2018). These frequencies resonate deeply with the body's cells, creating healing vibrations that support emotional wellness.

  Solfeggio frequencies are thought to resonate deeply with our energy fields, and studies have shown that exposure to these frequencies can reduce stress, increase clarity and promote emotional healing. These sounds align with your body's energy fields and DNA, promoting emotional, physical and spiritual healing on a deep, cellular level.

- 417 Hz—Facilitating Change and Releasing Stuck Energy
- 528 Hz—DNA Repair, Transformation, Love and Miracles
- 174 Hz—Pain Relief and Deep Healing
- 852 Hz—Spiritual Clarity and Alignment
- 396 Hz—Releasing Fear and Guilt for Emotional Freedom
- 963 Hz—Awakening and Expanding Consciousness
- 7.83 Hz—Earth's Harmony (Schumann Resonance) for Grounding
- 741 Hz—Emotional Expression and Clarity
- 639 Hz—Harmonizing Relationships and Connection
- 432 Hz—Universal Frequency for Inner Peace
- 285 Hz—Cellular Repair and Tissue Regeneration
- 1000–10,000 Hz—Tinnitus Relief and Sound Healing

Scan the QR Code to tune into
Team Luke's Sound Medicine Healing Playlist.

Some aspects to keep in mind while listening to these:

- Listen on a low volume as a background sound.
- Loop to experience the maximum benefits.
- Drink adequate water before and after these tones.
- Headphones are optional.

Play them in the background while you work, relax or meditate. Use apps and playlists dedicated to these healing frequencies.

***Disclaimer:** Do not listen to these frequencies while driving or operating heavy machinery. Avoid overusing these frequencies at a high volume; take regular intervals between each listen.*

Sound healing frequencies are not a replacement for medical treatment. Always make an informed choice. Keep your healthcare provider in the loop before trying anything new, especially if you have a medical condition or are on medications.

The Science of Sound and Emotional Healing

- A study published in *Frontiers in Neuroscience* explored the effects of sound meditation and showed that participants experienced significant reductions in tension, anger and fatigue (Chen et al., 2024). Moreover, sound-based therapies, like music therapy, have been shown to help patients with PTSD, supporting emotional balance through the soothing effects of certain frequencies in studies published in *Psychology and Psychotherapy* (Carr et al., 2012).

- Sound waves enter the body, interact with our energy fields and synchronize brainwaves. In doing so, they create a sense of inner calm, which is essential for emotional healing. The gentle vibrations produced by various sound healing techniques help to reset the nervous system, promoting a state of relaxation that allows emotional blockages to be released.

One of my clients, Sarah, had been struggling with chronic anxiety for years. We incorporated sound healing—specifically, Tibetan singing bowls—into her lifestyle protocol. After a few sessions, Sarah reported feeling more relaxed and centred than she had in years. The constant 'buzz' of anxiety was quietened, and her sleep improved dramatically.

Another example is Jonathan, a man who had suffered from grief and emotional blockages after losing a loved one. He began attending regular gong baths, and over time, he described the experience as a release. The sound waves allowed him to let go of emotions he had been holding onto, and he emerged from the sessions feeling lighter and more at peace.

Sound is a powerful healer that has been used for centuries, and modern science is now catching up with what ancient traditions knew all along.

By making sound healing a part of your daily routine, you can reduce anxiety, promote emotional balance and support overall well-being. Embrace this gentle yet powerful tool, and allow the vibrations of sound to guide you towards greater peace and harmony in your life.

74

Focused Reading for Relaxation

One powerful, often overlooked, method to relax and move from SNS to PNS is focused reading. You may have read all about the benefits of reading and its incredible power on the mind. But what is focused reading? Think of reading, but 10x times more powerful and immersive.

Engaging in deep, concentrated reading can shift your body from the fight-or-flight response to the rest-and-digest mode. How? Let's explore.

The Science Behind Focused Reading and the PNS

Focused reading can activate the PNS by allowing the mind to concentrate on a single, calming activity. This deep engagement shifts the brain into a state of flow.

Research conducted at the University of Sussex found that reading for just 6 minutes can reduce stress by up to 68 per cent (Lewis, 2009). Reading outperformed other relaxation methods, such as listening to music or taking a walk, when it came to reducing stress levels.

When you immerse yourself in a book, especially one that captures your interest, your mind is occupied with the narrative or information, which reduces the cognitive load from other stressors. This singular focus helps quieten the mind, thus encouraging relaxation.

Reading at a steady pace, especially silently, can naturally slow your breathing and heart rate, both of which are indicators of PNS activation. This is similar to the effects of meditation, where focused attention and deep breathing are used to induce relaxation.

Engaging with characters and stories fosters empathy, broadens your perspective, reduces stress and promotes a sense of connection.

According to a 2013 study published in *Science*, reading literary fiction enhances the 'theory of mind'—the ability to understand others' mental states, emotions and intentions (Kidd and Castano, 2013). This process helps improve empathy, emotional regulation and interpersonal skills, which are crucial for mental well-being. Improved empathy and emotional processing are associated with lower levels of anxiety and depression, better emotional regulation and stronger relationships, all of which are key aspects of mental health.

Bibliotherapy as a Tool for Managing Depression and Anxiety

A 1991 study in the *Journal of Independent Social Work* explores the therapeutic use of books and reading materials for mental health. Self-help books, especially those focusing on cognitive-behavioural approaches, have been shown to significantly reduce symptoms of depression and anxiety (Pardeck, 1991).

Another 2018 meta-analysis in *Neuropsychiatric Disease and Treatment* reviewed bibliotherapy's effectiveness in treating depression and anxiety in children and adolescents. It found that focused reading of cognitive-behavioural materials significantly reduced symptoms of depression and anxiety (Yuan et al., 2018).

In a 1997 study in *Clinical Gerontologist,* focused reading was used as a treatment for older adults with disability experiencing depression and loneliness. The results showed that regular engagement in reading led to a reduction in depressive symptoms and helped alleviate feelings of isolation (Landreville and Bissonnette, 1997).

Embracing the Power of Focused Reading

Choose the Right Book

- **Fiction:** Novels, short stories or poetry that captivate your imagination can be great for relaxation.
- **Non-Fiction:** If you prefer non-fiction, opt for light, inspirational or self-help books that encourage positivity and mindfulness.
- **Genres:** Consider genres like fantasy, romance or historical fiction, which allow you to escape into different worlds and times.

Create a Relaxing Environment

- Find a cosy spot where you can sit or lie down comfortably. A soft chair, a bed or a hammock can be ideal.
- Use soft, warm lighting to create a soothing atmosphere. Avoid harsh, bright lights.
- If you enjoy background noise, consider playing soft, instrumental music or nature sounds at a low volume.

Set a Reading Routine

- Set aside a specific time each day for reading, such as before bed or during a quiet afternoon.
- Make sure this time is free from interruptions, turning off your phone or notifications to stay focused.

Mindful Reading

- Take your time with each page, savouring the words and allowing yourself to engage with the story or content fully.

- Practise deep breathing while reading to enhance relaxation. Inhale deeply, hold for a few seconds and exhale slowly.
- If reading fiction, try to visualize the scenes in your mind, immersing yourself in the story.

Reflect and Journal

- After reading, take a few minutes to reflect on what you've read. Consider how it made you feel and what thoughts it sparked.
- Write down your thoughts, favourite quotes or any insights. This can deepen your relaxation and connection to the material.

Focused reading for relaxation can become a cherished part of your self-care routine, helping you unwind and recharge.

Want to Take This a Step Further?

Listen to the audiobook while reading the text simultaneously. This form of immersive reading offers benefits beyond stress relief.

- Engaging both the visual and auditory senses helps reinforce information. The brain processes the same material in two different ways, leading to better understanding and memory retention.
- Listening and reading together allows you to catch nuances in the text that might be missed if only reading or listening. This is especially useful for complex or dense material.
- Listening to an audiobook while reading the text can anchor your attention, making it easier to maintain focus and enter a state of flow.
- Combining reading with listening creates a richer, more engaging multisensory experience, making the story or content more immersive and enjoyable.

- The tone and pace of a good narrator can add a soothing quality to the reading experience, helping to further slow your heart rate and promote relaxation. The narrator's voice can convey emotions, tone and accents that might be less evident in text alone, bringing characters and scenes to life in a more vivid way.
- The combined sensory input can help maintain your attention on the material, reducing the likelihood of daydreaming or getting distracted.
- Audiobooks set a consistent reading pace, which can help you stay focused, especially if you tend to skim or rush through text when reading silently.
- Encountering new words in both spoken and written form can enhance your vocabulary, as you're more likely to remember the word and its correct usage. Hearing words while seeing them in print helps improve pronunciation, especially for unfamiliar words or names. This is particularly beneficial for language learners.
- For individuals with dyslexia or other reading difficulties, following along with the text while listening can improve comprehension and reduce frustration.

Focused reading is more than just a way to pass the time; it is a scientifically backed method to shift your body into a state of relaxation by activating the PNS.

Whether you're seeking stress relief or just a deeper connection with your favourite books, this practice offers a simple, yet effective, solution. Adding an audiobook to the mix can elevate the experience. So, the next time you feel stressed, consider picking up a book and letting the words lead you into a state of calm.

75

The Gut–Brain Axis

You've probably heard the phrase **'trust your gut.'** It turns out that this isn't just a saying; it's rooted in science. The gut is often called our 'second brain' because of its complex interactions with the brain and its significant role in our overall health. This gut–brain connection is a powerful dialogue that goes beyond digestion, influencing immunity, mood and even mental health.

I consider any protocol to address a gut condition incomplete if we fail to address the mental health of the person experiencing it. The gut–brain connection plays a pivotal role in how our digestive system responds to stress, anxiety and emotions. In our practice, our approach to managing any gut case includes breaking down their emotional patterns and assessing their mental well-being. It is why our Gut Care Programme involves a life coach or counsellor, who helps our patients understand the deep connection between their emotions and their gut, thus empowering them to heal from within.

How much can your gut influence your health? Let me give you a real-life example of one of my clients.

This person came to me with an autoimmune condition. She had chronic IBS, severe hairfall, dull skin and acne covering her face. She also experienced a constant burning sensation in her stomach. Despite undergoing various treatments, including antacids, an endoscopy, Ayurveda and homoeopathy, nothing seemed to alleviate her symptoms.

We put her on a holistic protocol, incorporating *ajwain* water, *jeera* concoctions, pranayama and deep breathing exercises, but her symptoms persisted. After spending about 45 minutes going over her entire life, what we uncovered was astonishing. She had endured childhood abuse, a lack of support from her parents when she reported it and deep emotional pain caused by her husband. Her inability to forgive those who hurt her had created an emotional burden she had been carrying for years. Only when we began to break that down and counsel her on how to navigate those years of hurt did her condition begin to see a change.

The unresolved emotional trauma and lack of forgiveness manifested in her physical symptoms, especially of her gut. Without addressing the mental and emotional wounds, no treatment—no matter how holistic—could fully help her.

Decoding the Gut–Brain Connection

Have you ever prepared for an important meeting or presentation for weeks, rehearsing your points, feeling ready, only to wake up the morning of the event with a knot in your stomach, a racing heart and queasiness? You might even feel an urgent need to run to the restroom.

Does this sound familiar?

This isn't just nerves playing tricks on you; it's your gut reacting to signals from your brain. Stress, anxiety and pressure don't just stay confined to your mind; they ripple through your body and land squarely in your gut. It's why you might lose your appetite, when stressed, or feel your stomach churn before a big event.

Now, imagine this happening regularly—not just for important events but also during daily life. This constant gut reaction to mental stress can lead to bloating, indigestion and more serious conditions like IBS. Your body's way of saying, 'Something isn't right,' shouldn't be ignored.

The Enteric Nervous System: Your Gut's Own Brain

The reason behind this powerful connection lies in a unique system called the enteric nervous system (ENS), often referred to as the gut's own brain. The ENS consists of around 100 million nerve cells that line the gastrointestinal tract from the oesophagus to the rectum. This network of neurons communicates directly with the brain via the gut–brain axis.

Through this axis, your gut and brain send chemical and neural signals back and forth. The health of one can greatly affect the other. Stress, for example, can slow digestion, cause bloating and change gut bacteria. Likewise, an imbalanced gut can send distress signals to the brain, affecting your mood and even leading to anxiety and depression.

Stress, the Gut and the Nervous System

Your nervous system operates in two primary modes: the SNS, or 'fight-or-flight' mode, and the PNS, often called the 'rest-and-digest' mode. In today's fast-paced world, many of us spend too much time within the SNS, where stress hormones, like cortisol, are released.

Short bursts of cortisol during stressful situations can give you energy and focus, but chronic stress disrupts digestion and compromises gut health. Cortisol diverts energy away from 'non-essential' functions like digestion to deal with the perceived threat. Over time, chronic stress can lead to increased intestinal permeability, often called leaky gut, which allows harmful bacteria and toxins to enter the bloodstream, causing inflammation.

When we shift from the SNS to the PNS, we allow the body to rest, digest and repair itself. This transition is crucial for not only your mental health but also the health of your gut and immune system. The key is learning to shift from 'fight-or-flight' to 'rest-and-digest' more frequently.

What Does Science Say?

- **Stress and Gut Microbiome:** A study published in *Current Opinion in Behavioral Sciences* found that stress alters gut bacteria, leading to inflammation, digestive issues and a weakened immunity (Madison and Kiecolt-Glaser, 2019). This shows that stress not only affects the brain but also changes the gut's microbial landscape, creating a two-way dialogue.

- **Gut–Brain Axis and Mental Health:** Research published in *Brain, Behavior, and Immunity* has shown a strong correlation between gut microbiome diversity and mental health (Kraaij et al., 2023). This particular study shows how children with altered gut microbiome compositions were more likely to show emotional and behavioural problems. Individuals with more diverse gut microbiota showed lower levels of anxiety and depression, illustrating how gut health affects the brain and mood.
- **Leaky Gut and Autoimmunity:** Studies from *Food Science and Nutrition* highlight how chronic stress and poor gut health can lead to a 'leaky gut'. The study suggests that when the gut barrier is compromised, it increases the risk of autoimmune conditions, like inflammatory bowel disease (IBD), and even neurological issues such as Parkinson's disease (Liang, Saunders, and Sanossian, 2023).

Simple Ways to Shift from SNS to PNS

The good news is that we can take control of this powerful gut–brain connection. By engaging the PNS and nourishing our gut, we can enhance both physical and mental health.

Here are some simple, effective tips:

- Have a fibre-rich plate. Incorporate plenty of fruits, vegetables and whole grains to feed your gut's beneficial bacteria. Fibre supports digestion and helps keep the gut microbiome in balance.
- Fermented foods like yoghurt, sauerkraut, kimchi and kefir are packed with probiotics that increase

microbiome diversity. A diverse gut microbiome is linked to better immune function and mental health.

- Incorporate breathing exercises. Whether it's 4–7–8, or diaphragmatic/deep belly breathing, practising these can help you relax, reduce cortisol levels and improve digestion. This is particularly helpful when you feel anxious or stressed.
- One of the practices I love doing every morning is sunshine breath. Sit or stand facing natural light. Inhale for five counts, lift your arms, hold for two counts and then exhale for six counts, while lowering your arms. Repeat for 3 minutes.
- Taking just 5–10 minutes a day to meditate can also improve gut health. Studies show that mindfulness helps regulate the gut–brain axis by reducing cortisol and promoting a healthy microbiome.
- Certain yoga poses engage the PNS and promote relaxation. Try Child's Pose *(Balasana)* to soothe the gut, Cat-Cow Stretch *(Marjaryasana-Bitilasana)* to ease tension, and Bridge Pose *(Setu Bandhasana)* to relieve stress.
- Aim for 7–9 hours of sleep per night to support gut and brain health. Lack of sleep disrupts the microbiome and increases stress. Establish a calming bedtime routine, dim the lights and avoid screens before bed to optimize your sleep.
- Regular movement promotes gut health by improving circulation, reducing stress and supporting digestion. Activities like walking, cycling or yoga can improve the diversity of gut bacteria and reduce inflammation.
- Slow down. Chew your food thoroughly. Because digestion begins in your mouth. Avoid distractions like phones or TV while eating. Eating mindfully allows your body to engage in the digestion process fully, supporting both gut and mental health.

The Bigger Picture: Gut Health for Mental Health

Understanding and nurturing the gut–brain connection empowers you to take control of your health from the inside out. The gut isn't just the body's control centre for digestion; it's also the key to immunity, mental health and overall well-being. By shifting from the sympathetic to the parasympathetic mode, we can ensure that our bodies are thriving, both mentally and physically.

So, the next time you feel anxious, stressed or mentally drained, remember that your gut is listening. By caring for your gut with wholesome foods, managing stress and paying attention to your body's signals, you can create a foundation of health that benefits every part of your life.

Your gut—and your mind—will thank you for it.

Case Studies

- **Diabetes—Sarah's Journey**
  Sarah, a forty-five-year-old mother of two, was diagnosed with Type-2 diabetes. The hectic pace of her life, juggling work and family responsibilities, often left her feeling overwhelmed. Constant stress may lead to unhealthy eating habits and neglecting exercise.
  One day, after a particularly stressful incident at work, Sarah experienced a significant spike in her blood sugar levels. Frustrated, she decided to take control of her health.
  Sarah began integrating mindfulness meditation into her daily routine. She dedicated just 10 minutes each morning to focus on her breath, which allowed her to reset her emotional state. Additionally, Sarah started incorporating yoga twice a week, which not only helped relieve stress but also connected her with a community that supported her health journey.
  As months passed, her blood sugar levels stabilized, and her doctor noted a remarkable improvement. Sarah felt empowered, learning that slowing down and managing her stress was just as crucial as medication and diet.

- **Cancer—Guruprasad's Battle**
  At fifty-five, Guruprasad faced the diagnosis of Stage II prostate cancer. Following treatment, he found the emotional toll exhausting. Stress from the uncertainty about his health led to insomnia and feelings of hopelessness.

Seeking solace, Guruprasad joined a local support group for cancer survivors. Sharing his fears and listening to others' journeys helped him alleviate much of his emotional burden. He also picked up painting, a hobby he had abandoned years ago. This creative outlet kept him engaged and focused, distracting him from stressful thoughts.

With his newfound calm, Guruprasad began to visualize his healing through meditation. He envisioned his body battling cancer cells, which fostered a sense of empowerment. Over time, Guruprasad noticed that his scans showed reduced tumour activity. He realized that while medical treatments were vital, managing emotional stress played a key role in his recovery.

- **Obesity—Lisa's Transformation**

  Lisa had struggled with her weight for years, linking her emotional eating to her busy lifestyle and the constant pressure to excel at work. After hitting a breaking point, she decided to seek help.

  Lisa enrolled in a weight management programme and also emotional wellness workshops. Here, she learnt to differentiate between physical hunger and emotional cravings, which was a revelation for her. She implemented journalling, writing down her feelings and triggers, which helped her to recognize stress-induced eating patterns.

  She also started attending Zumba classes, where she met friends who celebrated small victories with her. As Lisa learnt to manage her stress through community and self-awareness, she gradually lost weight and regained her self-esteem, realizing the importance of being calm and centred in her life.

- **Autoimmune Issues—Mark's Experience**

  Mark was diagnosed with rheumatoid arthritis at forty. The chronic pain and fatigue made him irritable and stressed, affecting his relationships and work.

Desperate for relief, he researched and discovered the connection between stress and autoimmune diseases. Mark began a regular meditation practice, focusing on body awareness and acknowledging his pain without judgement. He also explored Tai Chi, which combined movement with mindfulness and helped him release tension.

Within months, Mark reported reduced pain levels, and his inflammatory markers improved. His doctors noted a positive shift in his overall health. Mark's journey taught him that a calm mind could positively influence his autoimmune response.

- **Skin Issues—Trish's Recovery**

  Trish had dealt with severe acne for years, leaving her feeling self-conscious and anxious. Dermatologists prescribed treatments, but nothing seemed to work long-term.

  Determined to find a solution, she researched the impact of stress on skin health. Trish adopted a daily skincare routine that emphasized gentle care and hydration, but more importantly, she started prioritizing self-care, which included long walks in nature and practising gratitude.

  As her stress levels decreased, so did her breakouts. Trish also began participating in group therapy, which made her feel supported and less alone. In time, her skin cleared significantly, revealing that managing emotional stress was illuminating her path to healing.

- **Hair Issues—Nirvaan's Reflection**

  Nirvaan, at thirty-eight, began losing his hair and attributed it to genetics and work-related stress. The emotional weight of the situation compounded his stress, leading to increased hair loss and lower self-confidence.

  Through research, Nirvaan learnt that stress could exacerbate hair loss. He sought therapy to address his underlying anxiety and began practising deep breathing exercises. Engaging in physical activities, such as cycling and swimming, allowed him to channel his stress constructively.

With time, Nirvaan noticed that by managing his stress and focusing on his well-being, the rate of his hair loss slowed. More importantly, he regained confidence, realizing that emotional calmness was critical in facing life's challenges.

- **Gut Issues—Rachel's Healing**

  Rachel suffered from IBS, which caused her considerable discomfort and emotional distress. Triggered by stress, her symptoms led to a vicious cycle where anxiety exacerbated her gut issues.

  Rachel consulted a nutritionist who introduced her to gut-health-promoting foods and techniques like mindful eating. She also embraced yoga to focus on relaxation and stress release.

  Incorporating these practices helped Rachel become more attuned to her body. Over several months, her symptoms lessened significantly, demonstrating how managing stress was key to her gut health recovery.

- **Hormonal Issues—Alice's Balance**

  At fifty, Alice experienced extreme hormonal fluctuations during menopause, leading to bouts of irritability, anxiety and fatigue. Feeling out of control, she took it upon herself to seek a holistic approach to manage her symptoms.

  Alice began attending workshops focusing on stress management and hormone balance. She learned the importance of regular exercise, adequate sleep and healthy nutrition. Mindful breathing became a daily practice to alleviate anxiety and restore calmness.

  Gradually, as Alice implemented these lifestyle changes and learned to manage her stress, her symptoms improved dramatically. She felt empowered by her body's transformation, realizing how intertwined emotional health and physical wellness truly are.

Acknowledgements

Special thanks to **Tyanna Brooklyn Coutinho, Natashya Phillips, and my wonderful family and friends** for their constant understanding and support.

To all the **incredible individuals, readers and well-wishers around the globe**—your trust, commitment to better health and heartfelt encouragement remind us why this work matters every single day.

To **Taarika** and **Jovita,** who have been an inseparable part of all my books. *The Calm Prescription* is not just a book—it's a marvel born out of years of observation, reflection and experience. A blend of science and real-life transformational stories.

To every **doctor and medical expert** we've had the privilege to collaborate with, thank you for believing in the power of integrative and lifestyle medicine. For daring to talk about how emotional wellness is often the missing puzzle piece in health.

To our **clients**, you are our greatest teachers. From every consultation, every breakthrough, every struggle and every victory, we've seen how the body listens and responds in a state of calm, and how chronic stress can disrupt even the most perfect lifestyle. These real-time insights are what shaped the principles in this book, and for that, we are deeply grateful.

To **Team Luke**—thank you for standing strong with us through every season. What you do isn't easy: navigating time zones, conditions, emotions and cultures, all while managing your own personal journeys. You walk the talk with grace and grit. Your empathy, calm and commitment to make a difference is the heartbeat of our vision.

To **Milee and the entire Penguin Random House India team**, thank you for believing in the power of our message and backing it with your heart and hands.

Special gratitude to **Sister B.K. Shivani, Gurudev Sri Sri Ravi Shankar, Dr Jonathan Fisher, Vidya Balan, Ankur Warikoo, Tamannaah Bhatia, Dr Anil Kohli, Dr Nihar Mehta, Dr Sonali Kohli, Dr Ganesh Nagarajan, Dr Aashish Contractor, Dr Maulik Parekh, Taylor Elizabeth, Dr Hansaji Yogendra, Dr Anil D'Cruz, Dr Sachin Trivedi, Dr Nozer Sheriar, Dr Amit Maydeo, Dr Sudhir Pillai, Vispy Kharadi** and **Dr (Col) Prakash Dave**—your faith, time and advance praise for this book are deeply cherished.

To anyone who picks this book up, may it be a gentle reminder that the prescription we most often overlook—calm—could be the most powerful one we hold.

With gratitude,
Luke Coutinho

For references, please scan this QR code.